"This bold and provocative new book draws on psychoanalysis to call into doubt many of the fundamental and common-sense assumptions about how censorship works and what it is for. William Simms contests standard accounts of these trials as straightforwardly repressive or enlightened. Instead, he shows how the outcome of the trials was much less important than the modes of desire and enjoyment that the trials articulated, and the mechanisms exercised by literary criticism and other discourses to regulate desire and enjoyment. *Obscenity, Psychoanalysis and Literature* is a work of great fluency and genuine invention."

— *Peter Buse, Dean of the School of the Arts at the University of Liverpool*

OBSCENITY, PSYCHOANALYSIS AND LITERATURE

Obscenity, Psychoanalysis and Literature offers a fascinating psychoanalytic reading of four landmark obscenity trials involving the texts of D. H. Lawrence and James Joyce. By tracing the legal histories of Lawrence and Joyce, from censorship to their eventual redemption and transformation into champions of sexual freedom, the book draws a narrative of changing legal, literary and cultural investments.

The book examines the four trials of these authors in detail to show how the literary text can function as a symbol of both life and death and the political uses of figuring them as such. Taking a psychoanalytic perspective, we can see how this narrative of sexual repression to sexual liberation may itself be an emergent form of the superego imperative to enjoy and consume. Through close readings of trial transcripts and archival documents, this book helps elucidate the fantasies operating throughout the trials: the unquestioned assumptions of the nature of sexuality, gender, drugs and truth. It demonstrates with clarity how, through its attempt to suppress the sexual, the law confronts its own nature as language and in doing so troubles the distinctions between law, literature and desire that it usually wishes to protect.

Offering a uniquely psychoanalytic account of the obscenity trials of these authors, this text will be of great interest to scholars from across the fields of psychoanalysis, law and literature.

William Simms received the President's Doctoral Scholar Award from the University of Manchester, UK, where he completed his Ph.D. He is an interdisciplinary researcher, interrogating the intersections between literary, legal and psychoanalytic discourses.

The Lines of the Symbolic in Psychoanalysis Series

Series Editor: Ian Parker, Manchester Psychoanalytic Matrix

Psychoanalytic clinical and theoretical work is always embedded in specific linguistic and cultural contexts and carries their traces, traces which this series attends to in its focus on multiple contradictory and antagonistic 'lines of the Symbolic'. This series takes its cue from Lacan's psychoanalytic work on three registers of human experience, the Symbolic, the Imaginary and the Real, and employs this distinctive understanding of cultural, communication and embodiment to link with other traditions of cultural, clinical and theoretical practice beyond the Lacanian symbolic universe. The Lines of the Symbolic in Psychoanalysis Series provides a reflexive reworking of theoretical and practical issues, translating psychoanalytic writing from different contexts, grounding that work in the specific histories and politics that provide the conditions of possibility for its descriptions and interventions to function. The series makes connections between different cultural and disciplinary sites in which psychoanalysis operates, questioning the idea that there could be one single correct reading and application of Lacan. Its authors trace their own path, their own line through the Symbolic, situating psychoanalysis in relation to debates which intersect with Lacanian work, explicating it, extending it and challenging it.

Obscenity, Psychoanalysis and Literature
Lawrence and Joyce on Trial
William Simms

Lacan, Mortality, Life and Language
Clinical and Cultural Explorations
Berjanet Jazani

Psychoanalysis Under Nazi Occupation
The Origins, Impact and Influence of the Berlin Institute
Laura Sokolowsky

For more information about this series, please visit: https://www.routledge.com

OBSCENITY, PSYCHOANALYSIS AND LITERATURE

Lawrence and Joyce on Trial

William Simms

Routledge
Taylor & Francis Group
LONDON AND NEW YORK

First published 2022
by Routledge
2 Park Square, Milton Park, Abingdon, Oxon OX14 4RN

and by Routledge
605 Third Avenue, New York, NY 10158

Routledge is an imprint of the Taylor & Francis Group, an informa business

British Library Cataloguing-in-Publication Data
A catalogue record for this book is available from the British Library

Library of Congress Cataloging-in-Publication Data
Title: Obscenity, psychoanalysis and literature : Lawrence and Joyce on trial / William Simms.
Description: Abingdon, Oxon ; New York : Routledge, 2022. | Series: Lines of the symbolic in psychoanalysis | Includes bibliographical references and index. | Summary: "Obscenity, Psychoanalysis and Literature offers a fascinating psychoanalytic reading of four landmark obscenity trials involving the texts of D. H. Lawrence and James Joyce. By tracing the legal histories of Lawrence and Joyce, from censorship to their eventual redemption and transformation into champions of sexual freedom, the book draws a narrative of changing legal, literary and cultural investments. Offering a uniquely psychoanalytic account of the obscenity trials of these authors, this text will be of great interest to scholars from across the fields of psychoanalysis, law and literature"—Provided by publisher.
Identifiers: LCCN 2021013886 (print) | LCCN 2021013887 (ebook) | ISBN 9781032064833 (hardback) | ISBN 9781032064864 (paperback) | ISBN 9781003202509 (ebook)
Subjects: LCSH: Joyce, James, 1882–1941—Criticism and interpretation. | Lawrence, D. H. (David Herbert), 1885–1930—Criticism and interpretation. | Law and literature—History—20th century. | Psychoanalysis and literature—History—20th century. | Trials (Obscenity)—History—20th century. | LCGFT: Literary criticism.
Classification: LCC PR6019.O9 Z7956 2022 (print) | LCC PR6019.O9 (ebook) | DDC 823/.912—dc23
LC record available at https://lccn.loc.gov/2021013886
LC ebook record available at https://lccn.loc.gov/2021013887

ISBN: 978-1-032-06483-3 (hbk)
ISBN: 978-1-032-06486-4 (pbk)
ISBN: 978-1-003-20250-9 (ebk)

DOI: 10.4324/9781003202509

Typeset in Bembo
by codeMantra

CONTENTS

SERIES PREFACE

Fantasy and power are always at stake when psychoanalysis encounters the law, and it has often been the case in the popular imagination, and sometimes in the institutions that regulate what it is healthy and normal to think and feel about ourselves and others, that psychoanalysis itself poses a threat to the law, signaling that something of fantasy may subvert and perhaps even break through the carapace of order. While psychoanalysis in the clinic utilizes and appeals to some notion of law, most notably in its specifications what a path through the Oedipal drama might look like for each individual subject and what kind of power that subject must acknowledge as it enters language and society, the symbolic order, it has often found itself cast on the other side of the equation, as avatar of fantasy that the law then tries to hold in check.

Nowhere is this more the case than when the fantasy that psychoanalysis speaks for is explored in literature, and when fantasy is re-cast by the law as something obscene. There is no outside of this game, no metalanguage that can speak of it objectively, and the kind of writing that speaks of subjectivity, 'literature' is treated as something dangerous when it spills beyond conventional limits of what should be written about in decent society.

That which psychoanalysis speaks of and for must, of its nature, be understood by the law as 'obscenity', but the contradictory meshwork of legal procedures by which obscenity can be licensed or prohibited, and the limits within which it can be spoken and written about, by whom and for what kind of audience, has changed over time. William Simms traces the way respectable authors and corruptible readers have been defined in key trials concerning what are now considered canonical literary texts by D. H. Lawrence and James Joyce. He shows how fantasy bears on the nature of something unbidden and untamable in the texts of these writers, something Lacan specified as 'jouissance', deadly pleasure beyond what can be countenanced by the pleasure principle, and by the law that governs it. The discourses of literature and law are tangled together in such a way that manifests not only representations of sexual pleasure – the ostensible target of legal action – but also of race, racism and class, class contempt which is reconfigured as something unspeakable, almost as contempt of court.

This is a book suffused with enjoyment, it is to be enjoyed, and it goes beyond what we might imagine of the law and what it symbolizes for us to encounter something beyond literature that structures how literature is contained, made readable.

Psychoanalytic clinical and theoretical work circulates through multiple intersecting antagonistic symbolic universes. This series opens connections between different cultural sites in which Lacanian work has developed in distinctive ways, in forms of work that question the idea that there could be single correct reading and application. The Lines of the Symbolic in Psychoanalysis series provides a reflexive reworking of psychoanalysis that transmits Lacanian writing from around the world, steering a course between the temptations of a metalanguage and imaginary reduction, between the claim to provide a god's eye view of psychoanalysis and the idea that psychoanalysis must everywhere be the same. And the elaboration of psychoanalysis in the symbolic here grounds its theory and practice in the history and politics of the work in a variety of interventions that touch the real.

Ian Parker
Manchester Psychoanalytic Matrix

INTRODUCTION

The sovereign rights of *jouissance*

From the mid-19th century up until the mid-20th century, British and American law courts took a much more direct and sustained role in policing literary texts. Of course, censorship of literary production has been a constant historical fact, and I will be making no attempt to claim this period of time as exceptional in that regard. However, the justifications for, and manner of, policing these texts points towards a specific cultural and historical investment in representations of sexuality. Sexually explicit material had been previously policed by the law courts of England but was part of a larger corpus of seditious materials including religious and political documents deemed potentially damaging to the sovereign power of the nation. The renewed investment in sexuality, the manner in which the sexuality of text becomes a political matter for the law, signifies a shift in power structures from a sovereign investment in maintaining power towards a biopolitical investment in managing populations. With this book, I wish to present a historical narrative through four case studies that details the emergence of this power structure and its transformation and mutation over time. By reading four trials of literary texts, beginning in 1915 and ending in 1960, I hope to show how the understanding of the literary text shifted from a potentially seditious threat to public health to an ally of biopolitical management during this period.

Michel Foucault argues in *The History of Sexuality* that the 19th century witnessed a transition away from a sovereign conception of power which focused on the right to kill to take away the life of a subject. Sovereign power, Foucault argues, 'was essentially a right of seizure: of things, time, bodies, and ultimately life itself; it culminated in the privilege to seize hold of life in order to suppress it'.[1] The 18th and 19th centuries saw, according to Foucault's narrative, the introduction of a new form of power that seeks not to take life but 'whose highest

DOI: 10.4324/9781003202509

function was perhaps no longer to kill, but to invest life through and through'.[2] Life itself became the object of power, what Foucault terms 'biopower', and in this sense, the proliferation of obscenity trials is in keeping with power's newfound interest in the subject's sexual hygiene, a key site of biopolitical investment. But, according to Foucault, this shift also meant a depreciation of the law as the focal point of power: power was now dissipated into numerous disciplinary discourses, each acting according to their own norm, and through the intersection of these discourses, the biopolitical subject is produced. Whilst this book will maintain an emphasis on power's investment in the subject's sexuality as a locus of truth and object of surveillance, I also wish to argue for the continued status of the law as a primary means for the dissemination of power: even if the law is no longer the ultimate locus of power, it still functions as the means by which the truth claims of power are legitimated, and the subject's fantasy of an ordered and natural relation between power and truth is maintained: thus, the legal trial can be thought of as the process by which the multiple and sometimes contrary truth claims of power are both contested and legitimated.

By introducing the idea of fantasy as a means of bridging the gap between the discursive productions of power and the subject's perception of truth, I am bringing together the sometimes disparate discourses of biopolitics and psychoanalysis. In doing so, I hope to better delineate the manner in which biopolitics manages to remain and intensify and to identify the law as the ground upon which the competing truth claims of disciplinary discourses come to be decided upon and legitimated: the law is the means by which biopower presents itself as a consistent ideology.

My argument begins with two, interconnected, concerns: why is the law invested in sex and why is the law invested in literature? The fact that the law desires to police these two phenomena would seem to indicate a potentially seditious element operating in both. What brings these two concerns together, I believe, is their relation to *jouissance*.

Which in turn brings us to another difficult question: what exactly is *jouissance?* Like biopolitics, the psychoanalytic term *jouissance* will be doing a lot of work in this text, and it is best to attempt to detangle it as best as possible before beginning in earnest. To begin this analysis of the relationship between *jouissance* and the law, we will turn to Freud's 1913 text *Totem and Taboo*. Freud's text attempts to posit a universal origin of law and morality that takes into account the work of desire and the presence of the unconscious. Emphasizing the apparent universal presence within societies of totemic worship and a taboo against incest, Freud theorizes that this universality points towards a shared primordial event that took place before the law and leading to its emergence. Freud hypothesizes a violent and patriarchal form of life, wherein 'primeval man aboriginally lived in small communities, each with as many wives as he could support and obtain, whom he would have jealously guarded against all other men'.[3] This theory of a space before the law is not then lawless but governed by another law, under the auspices of a sovereign whose power consisted in his ability to enjoy and wherein enjoyment is figured as a zero-sum game: the primal father's enjoyment comes at the expense of the other males. This uneven distribution of enjoyment instilled in the patriarch's sons a desire to revolt against their violent father and claim what they felt was their right to enjoy:

> One day the brothers who had been driven out came together, killed and devoured their father and so made an end of the patriarchal horde. United, they had the courage to do and succeeded in doing what would have been impossible for them individually.[4]

If the previous libidinal economy of the primal father had been profoundly individualistic, this collective act by the brothers constitutes the creation of a social body bound by a collective identification as both brothers and victims of the father's prohibition. But in murdering the father and the act of incorporating his body through eating his body to gain access to his enjoyment, the sons betray a prior identification with the murdered father, an identification that the murder attempts to re-establish through the removal of the only barrier to it. Before the crime that instigates the law, then, there is at play in Freud's narrative an ambivalence wherein the collective identity that spurs the constitutive crime is itself a misidentification: fraternity and equality are themselves products of a frustrated identification with the law itself, the subject is then exterior to the law and by attempting access, as we shall see, only succeeds in confirming his exteriority.

This identification with the figure of the law is confirmed and repeated in the ritual of the totem meal in which the usurpation of the father and his incorporation by the sons is celebrated:

> The violent primal father had doubtless been the feared envied model of each one of the company of brothers: and in the act of devouring him they accomplished their identification with him, and each one of them acquired a portion of his strength. The totem meal, which is perhaps mankind's earliest festival, would thus be a repetition and a commemoration of this memorable and criminal deed.[5]

The new society instituted by the sons continues to return to this site of trauma and through the feast enjoys this ambivalence, wherein the identification with the father as well as his destruction is repeated. Every return thus constitutes a renewed destruction of the father and celebration of fraternity, wherein the father's former strength and potency is distributed among his sons. But this identification also produces anxiety in the sons, as, in death, the latent love felt for the father and the primary identification with him re-emerge in a sense of guilt. As Freud states:

> They hated their father, who presented such a formidable obstacle to their craving for power and their sexual desires; but they loved and admired him

> too. After they had got rid of him, had satisfied their hatred and had put into effect their wish to identify themselves with him, the affection which had all this time been pushed under was bound to make itself felt.[6]

The full violence of the act of identification is thus felt. In the enactment of this identification, that aims to erase the distinction between the subject and the other with whom he identifies, the death of the other no longer allows for the completion of this identification. The subject is thus, once again, alienated from their identification with the figure of the law. The sons' rebellion and usurpation of the father importantly fails to achieve its desired aims, and the totemic meal comes not to represent their success at taking the father's place and achieving a fair partitioning of the father's original enjoyment, but instead comes to stand for an attempt to regain what was lost in the act of killing the father: his apparently limitless enjoyment has not been passed on to the sons, and his absence is felt as a lack rather than a gain.

This failure, Freud argues, brings about a sense of guilt in the sons:

> This fresh emotional attitude must also have been assisted by the fact that the deed cannot have given complete satisfaction to those who did it. From one point of view it had been done in vain. Not one of the sons had in fact been able to put his original wish—of taking his father's place—into effect. And, as we know, failure is far more propitious for a moral reaction than satisfaction.[7]

By virtue of having to band together in order to claim the father's enjoyment, this enjoyment must, after his death, be shared among the sons. By ending the father's monopoly on enjoyment, their ability to enjoy that monopoly disappears with it. The potential for limitless enjoyment, one definition of *jouissance*, has died with the father. This loss marks the sons' failure too. This failure produces in them a sense of guilt, a desire for the father to return and, with him, the potential enjoyment that also died with him. This guilt thus signifies a dependency not upon the father himself but the enjoyment which he had come to represent to the sons.

An irony is also in play here. Only in death, in the father's own failure, would his domination over the sons be total. As Freud goes on to explain:

> The dead father became stronger than the living one had been [...].What had up to then been prevented by his actual existence was thenceforward prohibited by the sons themselves [...]. They revoked their deed by forbidding the killing of the totem, the substitute for their father; and they renounced its fruits by resigning their claim to the women who had now been set free.[8]

The living father had been proven impotent by his sons' insurrection against him. But, in death, the potency ascribed to him by the sons prior to his death and desired by the sons is lost. As a means of resurrecting the potential for this full enjoyment and, crucially, a semblance of order, the father is reincarnated in the form of fantasy. Fantasy, then, comes to protect the sons from anxiety and alleviate them from the trauma of their deed. Freud imagines the law as being born from a sense of guilt, a guilt produced by a desire for the impossible. The law, in this case, the taboo against incest and the killing of the totem animal, acts as the means to maintain the fantasy of the father, of a sovereign power who gives order to chaos. The father has transitioned from the father of the Real, an embodiment of destructive enjoyment, into the guarantor of the Symbolic.

But here, we've slipped into Lacan when we were supposed to be discussing Freud. These categories of Real, Symbolic and Imaginary are alien to Freud only inasmuch as they are never fully categorized in his texts, but their interplay, as Lacan is keen to point out, can be drawn out readily. A further analysis of this Lacanian distinction between the Real, Imaginary and Symbolic orders will be attempted later in this text, but for now, we can posit them as follows. The Symbolic order constitutes the domain of the signifier, which can be spoken or written word but can also any gesture that can be said to carry meaning. Subjects are first and foremost, for Lacan, speaking beings: language forms the crux of our relation to the world and our own identities. But, crucially, the signifier, for many reasons, I shall explore in depth later in this text, fails to complete its task of legislating for the subject's complete understanding and enjoyment of herself or the world. As such, the Imaginary order is required to suture this lack and appease the subject's discontents and frustration with the signifier. The Imaginary is thus the realm of fantasy, another key concept for this book and one I hope to show operative at the level of law in general and these trials specifically throughout. The Real, probably the most seductive and often misappropriated aspect of this triad, constitutes the repressed element of the interplay between the Imaginary and Symbolic. The Real is that which cannot be spoken by the signifier and is yet present in its movement, and it is that which fantasy attempts to veil and keep at an appropriate distance. It is worth stating that the Real does not represent a zone of truth in psychoanalysis as it can sometimes be understood. We are never looking directly for the Real of the subject nor does it constitute the truth of the world outside of language. Instead, the Real is the product of the enunciation of the signifier, that which is missed and yet must return in some form.

To put it simply, before returning to the discussion of Freud's text, the Symbolic is the realm of language, the Law, the sovereign and the father. The Imaginary is the realm of fantasy, identity and desire. The Real is the realm of disruption, the death drive and *jouissance*. Of course, in psychoanalysis, things are never so clear cut and I hope to complicate this relation by showing how these three orders interact in the form of the primal father in Freud's myth.

Primarily, I am concerned with Freud's depiction of the law as a shield against the unbearable and unstable *jouissance* of the primal father, as a means of producing and maintaining fantasmatic consistency and collective identity. This will be one understanding I will take of the term *jouissance*, a form of total enjoyment without limits, incommensurate with the signifier and, therefore, inherently transgressive. The law, according to Freud, originates in a traumatic encounter with *jouissance* which only a fantasmatic object-come-barrier can alleviate. It is the production and maintenance of that fantasy which is at work within legal discourse.

But, crucially missing from Freud's account of the law's origin is the role of sexual difference: what is woman's relation to the law? The women are figured as the cause of the brothers' jealousy against the father and the evidence of their crime. Both, before and after the event, the women are objects of enjoyment for the men. If the woman's initial relation to the primal father is an object possessed wholly by the father, the subsequent position is still as a commodity, only now under a regulated ownership between the brothers. So, in a sense, the duty to the father that emerges with his death also depends upon a regulation and management of women as objects of desire and a repression of women as desiring subjects. Feminine enjoyment can thus be figured as heterogeneous to the economy that emerges in relation to the duty to the father and thus a form of transgression that resists the law of the father. Thus, the law's investment in the name-of-the-father is concomitant with a desire to police femininity to ensure its place but also to police its boundaries. We have our first instance of interlocking and mutually dependent fantasies: ~~The~~ Law and ~~The~~ Woman.

The law, and the forms of fantasy it protects, requires sexual difference to be figured in a particular way for those fantasies to function. The law, in these trials, is invested in a conception of sexual difference that emphasizes the harmonious relations between male and female, with the male side distinctly privileged. This male privilege is maintained by a simultaneous fetishisization of ~~The~~ Woman and repression of feminine enjoyment. Key to the consistency of the benevolent father of law is a concomitant fantasy of ~~The~~ Woman. I will go into more detail on this fantasy figure of ~~The~~ Woman and how it differs from the lived experience of feminine subjects in my prologue to Part 1 of this book. This book will chart the manner in which the trials unconsciously testify to the labour required to maintain these various fantasmatic investments. The law thus requires a fantasy of harmonious sexual relations, a fantasy this thesis, following Lacan, will refer to as the fantasy of the sexual relation.

Before moving on to the gendered aspect of the law and psychoanalysis, it is worth asking the question as to why, at this particular historical moment, Freud felt the need to posit this hypothesis about the origins of law, and why such an origin needed to be posited in the first place. Eric Santner in his analysis of Freud's case study of Judge Schreber argues that the end of the nineteenth and the beginning of the 20th centuries constituted a historical 'crisis of investiture', wherein the very grounds of the law's legitimacy and its power, those very symbolic rights that Freud describes in *Totem and Taboo*, were being challenged. Expanding on the nature of these symbolic institutions and their power to bestow meaning for the subject, Santner argues that:

> the social and political stability of a society as well as the psychological "health" of its members would appear to be correlated to the efficacy

> of these symbolic operations—to what we might call their performative magic—whereby individuals "become who they are," assume the social essence assigned to them by way of names, titles, degrees, posts, honors, and the like.[9]

Santner's argument emphasizes the law as a linguistic institution dependent upon language to govern. It is through language that the law bestows on subjects an identity and rights. But, if we understand that the connection between the signifier and the reality, it is supposed to represent as sutured by fantasy, then these identities conferred by the law can be understood as contingent rather than essential. The 'performative magic' of the law that confers on the subject their very essence, what is in them more than themselves, is itself dependant on the subject believing that the law does not produce their identity but rather names what is already there. The subject is then libidinally invested in the law through this form of fantasy. An investiture crisis instigates the disintegration of the fantasmatic fabric through which the subject desires:

> an "investiture crisis" has the potential to generate not only feelings of extreme alienation, anomie, and profound emptiness, anxieties associated with absence; [...] a generalized attenuation of symbolic power and authority can be experienced as the collapse of social space and the rites of institution into the most intimate core of one's being. The feelings generated thereby are [...] anxieties not of absence and loss but of overproximity, loss of distance to some obscene and malevolent presence.[10]

The performative magic that allows symbolic rights to be perceived as essential qualities of the subject is itself a fiction held in place by fantasy. The crisis of investiture that Santner describes as taking place at the turn of the century corresponds to an increasing awareness of these symbolic fictions *as* fictions, that is, as having no essential grounds upon which their truth can be claimed beyond their own pronouncements. Crucially, this collapse of symbolic power results in the emergence of obscenity, a profoundly destructive and sexual form of enjoyment that threatens the subject's identity. This process will repeat itself throughout the trials analysed in this thesis: The failure of the Symbolic and the disintegration of fantasy results in the emergence of sex. Sex and truth will repeatedly come into conflict in these trials until, in the final trial, an attempt will be made to incorporate sex and its perceived power into these symbolic cultural practices.

It is to this problem of law as a fiction, grounded in nothing, but its own utterance and repetition that Freud's myth of the primal father aims to both explain and repair. Freud's myth is decidedly secular. It claims to be the empirical origin of all subsequent religious myths, but itself requires no divine intervention. Santner notes that this crisis of investiture partly resulted from the diminishing influence of religious institutions in Western Europe, thus rupturing one of the means by which subjects could ground their identity and organize their desire.[11] As well as displaying an absence of divine will, Freud's myth also lacks the event of a sovereign decision from which the law originates. The primal father, as sovereign, who in Carl Schmitt's definition is 'he who decides on the exception' is presented in Freud's narrative as ultimately impotent and unable to ground his decision in anything but violence towards the sons.[12] Violence is thus presented as the zero-level of the law, with the sovereign presented as the exception who is permitted to enjoy without limit. This intersection of *jouissance* and law, obscenity and truth, is ultimately untenable because it is felt by the sons to be a form of injustice and therefore illegitimate. A functioning law thus requires a minimal fantasmatic distance, a minimal level of buy in from the subject, in order to be perceived as legitimate. Without this distance, the law itself becomes stained by enjoyment, the presence of which disqualifies it as law and outs itself as fiction. Or, as Freud argues, 'Sexual desires do not unite men but divide them'.[13] Law in this conception must remain desexualized in order to act as an agent of social cohesion. This necessary renunciation of sexuality allows for the appearance of neutrality and the production of objective and reasoned decision making. Conversely, sex, as conceived by the law, is a threat to the law's existence which partly explains the law's investment in policing *jouissance*. Following this line of argument, a working definition of obscenity in relation to law can be posited: *obscenity is enjoyment out of place.*

Once enjoyment is found outside of its designated practices and discourses, the structures delineating those proper places to enjoy and the institutions that police those boundaries are themselves stained by the very force, *jouissance*, that they derive their identity from policing.

Furthermore, the origin of the law is neither the result of the sovereign decision of king nor deity, but rather the specific failure of the sovereign's discourse to coincide with the world and the lived experience of his subjects. The sons, by contrast, band together to enact the act of parricide and, following the political implications of the myth, regicide. In the aftermath of his death, each son refutes his own right to sovereignty, instead deferring this function to a fantasmatic figure. The law is thus depicted as requiring a specifically unconscious fiction underwriting its machinations in order to grant it legitimacy and distance itself from improper enjoyment. In Freud's writing, such an agency is given the name super-ego and functions as the subject's internalization of the paternal law; in Lacan, this agency functions at the level of language and culture as the Big Other, a fantasmatic guarantor of the Symbolic Order. A crisis of investiture would be a return of the repressed enjoyment operative within the law, the sadism of the superego and the recognition of the primal father's law of violence as the only grounds by which the law, shorn of its fictitious truth claims, can continue to govern: in short, the law is not natural, the Big Other does not exist. Freud's attempt to re-write the origin of the law emphasizes that this historical moment required Freud's intervention in lieu of traditional religious or political fictions. It speaks to the law's dependency upon fiction, a dependency that must be repressed in order for the law to produce the effect of truth. Fiction and sexuality then are the targets of the law's circumscription as a means of disavowing their presence in its own discourse.

Hearing the siren's silence

If the law is based upon a fiction that it must continually repress in order to produce a claim to truth, then literature functions as its obscene double: literature is that which admits to its status as fiction and yet, in spite of this fact is felt to speak truth. How literature can be perceived as both a threat to truth and as embodying the truth, as the law's uncanny double and as the law's ally, will be a key concern of this book. In order to better explain how I will approach the literary text and its relation to truth, I will briefly discuss a text by another writer contiguous this crisis of investiture and with a similar investment in the law's absent origins: Franz Kafka. In the short story 'The Silence of the Sirens', Kafka initiates another return to and re-writing of an originary event, but in this case, it is the beginning of the Western literary canon, Homer's *Odyssey*. In Homer's original, Odysseus, wanting to hear the siren's song, but not suffer the deadly consequences, ties himself to the mast of the ship. He is tempted and driven to the limit of madness by their song but, due to his cunning strategy, escapes death and gains the knowledge that no man before him had lived to possess and repeat.

Kafka's version of the myth begins by immediately infantilizing Ulysses and bringing into question his traditionally depicted cunning. Ulysses is presented as ignorant of the knowledge that is said to be possessed by 'all of the world', thereby reversing the traditional reading of Homer's text, wherein Odysseus's possession of and desire for knowledge privileges him above the other members of his crew, thus bestowing upon him heroic status.[14] In Kafka's version, what marks Ulysses as exceptional is his ignorance which allows him to enjoy an 'innocent elation over his little stratagem'.[15] And, it is precisely Ulysses' ignorance rather than his cunning, which saves him from the sirens and the death that they threaten.

The sirens are not only capable of a seductive song in Kafka's narrative but also a different weapon, their silence. Their song, although ultimately fatal, recognizes the male subject as the object of their desire. Their silence, however, would signify a refusal of the male as desirable and refusing his desire to gain knowledge of their secret essence: But more than this, their silence could also signify the absence of this secret knowledge upon which Ulysses bases his identity. This silence is supposed to produce a demand in the subject to know: 'Against the feeling of having triumphed over them by one's own strength, and the consequent exaltation that bears down everything before it, no earthly powers can resist'.[16] The sirens' silence thus invokes in the listener a will to mastery over the sirens which links both the desire to know with a violent desire to control in the listening subject: these desires are linked in the knowledge that to know the sirens' truth means death, the act of mastery over them results in the death of the subject who attempts to assert his vitality over them.

Lacan, critiquing Kant's example of the subject who would repress his sexual desires for a lover if fulfilling them would lead to his death, argues that, contrary to reason, 'no occasion precipitates certain people more surely toward their goal than one that involves defiance of or even contempt for the gallows'.[17] The certain death promised by the gallows, by the law, or here by the sirens, could then arouse in the subject an intensification the desire to know, with the will-to-knowledge being privileged over the will to live.

If the sirens can represent an opportunity to triumph over death, they also represent a desire for death. Renata Salecl in her discussions of Homer's sirens argues that '[t]he Sirens themselves were neither dead nor alive: they were creatures in between - the living dead.[...] [T]hey were, on the one hand, pure desire, and, on the other hand, pure death'.[18] They testify to the potential co-existence of death and desire and a potential complicity between the two. In this sense, they too, like the primal father of Freud's myth, embody a form of destructive enjoyment that is both immensely attractive to the male subject whilst also requiring a distance to be maintained. Thus, Odysseus's cunning in Homer's narrative, wherein he manages to achieve the perfect balance between knowledge of the siren's song without the fatal consequence, comes to also represent the positioning of the subject in the perfect distance from his own destructive *jouissance:* The chains of Odysseus allow him to enjoy the encounter with death without succumbing to it. The function of the chains in the myth is concomitant with the function of fantasy as it relates to the law, providing a means of enjoyment that in turn shields the subject from the *jouissance* at work within the law.

And this attenuation to the fantasmatic quality of the sirens' song is what we see at play, and subverted within, Kafka's retelling. Ulysses is saved not by his knowledge but precisely by his misunderstanding of the events. In Kafka's version, the sirens do not sing to Ulysses, but he 'did not hear their silence; he thought they were singing and that he alone did not hear them'.[19] What facilitates this misidentification is his pre-existing desire to resist their seduction which causes him to misread their gesticulations as their song. It is also this misidentification which engenders a reversal of the economy of desire seen in Homer's version. In Kafka's version, it is Ulysses who becomes the object of desire of the sirens. His seeming indifference to their seduction causes them to lose 'any desire to allure; all that they wanted was to hold as long as they could the radiance that fell from Ulysses' great eyes'.[20] The encounter with Ulysses' indifference transforms the sirens into desiring subjects, themselves seduced by the mystery of Ulysses. But this secret knowledge that motivates their desire, the text is keen to emphasize, is not a form of truth but an error, a fiction believed to be a truth: what allows Ulysses to survive is the fantasy of seduction.

Salecl contends that the Homer's myth of the siren's song depends upon the necessary omission of the song itself. We are not given access to this embodiment of *jouissance*, instead having to accept the retelling, presumably from Odysseus upon his return. The siren's song, by virtue of its seductive quality and the threat of death that this seduction entails, cannot be narrated. Thus, this song of absolute presence, of limitless and deadly enjoyment, must remain silent. According to Salecl, 'the Sirens put the listeners in touch with [...] the knowledge in the real, that knowledge which the listeners do not want to know anything about'.[21] It is knowledge of a potential outside of the symbolic fictions, beyond the signifier, whose advent would coincide with complete enjoyment without the mediation of the Symbolic. But, critically, this space does not exist before language, before the law, but is, rather, the effect of the law's imposition, an effect of speech:

> This kernel is not simply something prior to symbolization; it is also what remains: what is left over from, or, rather, the failure of symbolization. The Sirens' song is the real that has to be left out for the story of the *Odyssey* to achieve form. However, there is no song of the Sirens before the story of the *Odyssey*. The Sirens' song is thus, on the one hand, that which incites the *Odyssey* as narration, while, on the other hand, it is also that which results from this narration: its remainder, which cannot be recounted.[22]

It is this impossible knowledge, knowledge of the object or the self in its entirety, beyond the mediation of the signifier, that allows for signification as such. For meaning to emerge, a beyond language that holds the potential for complete meaning must be posited: the signifier aims at a form of truth beyond its own utterance just as the sovereign's decision bases itself upon grounds beyond violence. But, in this act of speech, something is always missed which leaves traces of this originary misrecognition, the misrecognition of the signifier for the thing itself, the sovereign for the law and the law for natural order. This beyond the signifier, a zone of truth and 'natural' order that exists before the law and to which the law attempts to return in the act of decision, is a fantasy.

The act of seduction, or its threat, is a necessary structural fantasy of the law itself. Odysseus in Homer's version is an illustration of the law-abiding citizen, who, despite temptation, stays on the right side of the law, remains in his position as leader, dedicated to returning to his wife: the fantasy of seduction allows for him to enjoy this inherent transgression without destroying the structures that allow for this enjoyment in the first place.

But here, Kafka deviates and, in doing so, acknowledges the degree to which literature, by virtue of its openness to its own fictionality, allows for two endings, two truths held simultaneously. In the first ending, Ulysses, because of his fortunate misrecognition of presence where there was absence, escapes death and confirms his symbolic role as leader and hero. These symbolic roles, products of an apparent natural order and upheld by the law, remain despite the reversal that takes place in the two narratives: The law, even if based on misrecognition, still functions as law as long as it believes this misrecognition to be the truth. But Kafka's story ends with the intervention of another narrative that restores Ulysses' cunning, but in doing so undermines the very foundations upon which a natural order is founded.[23] In this second version of events, Ulysses is fully aware of the Siren's silence but knowing full well the investment in the act of seduction needed to maintain his position as master to his men and in order to avoid punishment by the gods, performs the role of seducee. In the face of the sirens' silence, of an absolute absence in the place of absolute presence, Ulysses performs as if he is tempted by the secret knowledge they offer in order to maintain in the subjects who watch him the possibility of this knowledge.

The way in which I wish to approach the literary text in the following work is, like others have before me, through the metaphor of the siren's song. Not, however, the sirens of Homer who offer the fantasy of a knowledge in the real that can be attained, a fantasy that functions as the inherent transgression to the law itself. Instead, I will attempt, like Kafka's text asks its reader, to hear the text's silence and remain attentive to the undecidability of the literary text. By refusing the assumption that a literary text has a truth outside of its own language or offers access to a form of truth beyond itself, the labour and libidinal investments of the law and the literary critic become apparent. Fantasy is itself a form of perpetual work, it needs to be produced and maintained. Rather than viewing the narrative of these trials as beginning with a misidentification of the literary object towards a gradual understanding of the text's truth and value, I wish to put forth the case that each trial consists of a range of misidentifications, on the part of prosecution and defence, of the literary text in general and the specific texts of Joyce and Lawrence in particular. That a text can be understood as both an embodiment of death in one trial and life in another does not admit to an error in one trial and the truth in the other. This instead testifies to the text's refusal to accede to the law's will to truth, as a silence being spoken over and spoken for.

I seek here not to remedy erroneous legal understandings of the text and offer my own, truer, understanding of the text. Instead, I wish to analyse the forms of fantasy operative in each understanding of the literary text and, by doing so, elucidate the specific libidinal and ideological investments operative within these claims to truth. I'm concerned with what has to be added and what must be taken away from the text in order to claim its truth: this, I believe, is key to understanding the power relations at play within these trials and within culture at large, and, in the final two chapters, literary criticism's complicity with the work of power.

A knife that cuts both ways

Intervening between law and literature is another discourse that cannot be readily assimilated to either side: psychoanalysis. Much has been written about the affinity between psychoanalysis and literature, both in the sense of literature's influence and anticipation of psychoanalytic ideas as well as Freud's own attempts at analysis of literary texts. For writers such as Shoshana Felman and Jacques Derrida, this affinity bestows on psychoanalysis a subversive quality in relation to the law and thus offers a useful tool for critiquing the truth claims of the law. Other critics have seen in the discourse of psychoanalysis a means to critique gendered power: the work of feminist psychoanalysts such as Juliet Mitchell and Jacqueline Rose emphasize the degree to which the patriarchal power structures described by Freud are ultimately shown to have no essential or natural basis.

However, these readings and uses of psychoanalysis contrast with, another, more critical approach to psychoanalysis. The works of Michel Foucault, Gilles Deleuze, Felix Guattari, Simone de Beauvoir and Kate Millett emphasize the appropriation of psychoanalysis by disciplinary and patriarchal power structures in order to maintain and reproduce these structures. Psychoanalysis, here, is on the side of the law and has provided the means by which the law propagates itself, forcing subjects to obey the heteronormative sexual demands of patriarchy and providing essentialist narratives for criminal dissidence according to pathological sexual behaviour.

This book wishes to take these latter claims seriously whilst also attempting to demonstrate the clear value of psychoanalysis for the means of critique. I would like to argue that the unconscious, like literature, in its silence, cannot be spoken for with certainty, it lacks any definitive essence. As such, any claim to essential qualities must, necessarily, misidentify the discourse and tactically misread.[24] The cause of the appropriation of psychoanalysis by the law does not solely derive from a misreading of Freud, but is a possibility that the texts of Freud both encourage and deny. The relationship between the law and its transgression, between Totem and Taboo, is a key concern for psychoanalysis, and as evidenced by Freud's constant return to myths of the origins of law, one that can never be resolved.

This impasse is centred upon the status of knowledge in the psychoanalytic technique. The person thinking alongside psychoanalysis, either analyst or critic, is forced to encounter the difficulty of ever being sure of the grounds upon which claims to truth are based. Lacan, building upon Freud, is particularly attuned to this difference. In *Seminar XI*, he advances the claim that '[t]ruth is based only on the fact that speech, even when it consists of lies, appeals to it and gives rise to it'.[25] Truth is an effect of language and therefore unavoidable as long as we remain speaking-beings. Language itself could not function as the basis for intersubjective communication without the underlying fantasy of a correlation between the signifier and the world.

Psychoanalysis's attention to the operation of desire within language creates a wider conception of truth that remains attentive to this underlying fantasy of a correlation between language and world whilst still, unavoidably, partaking in it. What counts as truth in legal discourse and what can count as true in psychoanalysis are therefore drastically different. As a means of working through this dynamic between two radically different epistemologies, I will have recourse to Lacan's framing of the transference around a fantasy figure of 'the subject supposed to know'.[26] As well as being the means by which the subject structures his desire, this formation also takes the form of a demand upon the Other. It is to this demand that the analyst must respond by either performing the role of the master with access to knowledge or by attempting to explore what forms of desire are at play in the creation of this fantasy. Also at play here in Lacan's formulation is the production of the object of knowledge itself. The object of knowledge that the other withholds from the subject is also an object of desire and equally imbued with fantasmatic investment: take, for example, the analysand who deeply desires a diagnosis, a signifier under which she can identify and structure her desire. Here, the other is the analyst to whom that desire is directed and can fulfil her desire to know. Here, we have two formulations of fantasy; first, the object of desire, the name under which the analysand will be able to finally identify, and the figure of the analyst as the subject who has access to this fantasized truth but continues to conceal it from the subject.

The obscenity trials with which this thesis is engaged will be analysed so as to bring out the problematics of knowledge and fantasy, emphasizing the traces of investments and labour operative within: What this book attempts is not a counter narrative that claims hegemony over previous narratives of this period of legal and literary history, but rather to investigate the manner in which legal truth is produced and the fantasmatic grounds such truth requires. This is the difference in the types of knowledge being produced by science and psychoanalysis and also the forms of truth produced by the law and literature.

It is worth briefly exploring how and if such a reading can be performed. When engaging in a psychoanalytic critique of truth, certain methodological problems begin to emerge: To what extent does the critique of mastery, the attempt to destabilize established forms of power, end up re-establishing them? In other words, how does one critically evaluate a legal decision on the interpretation of a literary text and avoid replacing it with an equally decisive and final one? The problem here is the problem of the critic who, in the process of attacking the discourse of the master, however inadvertently, posits himself as a new master. And in the case of interpretations of trials, a critic who positions himself as a judge, one better equipped than the ones who came before.

Psychoanalysis, too, has struggled with this paradox. In many ways, psychoanalysis is a transgressive discourse, illegitimate and discredited by scientific discourse, scandalous in its implication of sexuality in all human behaviour, dirtying those most precious and innocent libidinal treasures and continuously rebelling against established truths. However, it is also a discourse that names these transgressions, taxonomizes subject positions and, in some cases, offers complete explanations of texts, phenomena and subjects.

Foucault, in his lecture series of 1974–1975, repeatedly draws attention to the ways in which psychiatric discourses have been co-opted by legal discourse in order to explain the actions of potential criminals to prove or disprove their guilt. What the introduction of expert testimony in the 19th century managed to achieve, according to Foucault, was

> a certain privilege vis-a-vis any other element of judicial proof. … [T]hey are … privileged judicial statements that include statutory presumptions of truth, presumptions that are inherent in them according to whom it is that states them. In short, they are statements with specific effects of truth

> and power: a sort of supralegality of certain statements in the production of judicial truth.[27]

What distinguishes the expert witness from any other testimony is his status, or rather the presumption of his status, as a master, and his access to the subject's truth. In a trial, an arena in which the status of the subject's truth is being contested, the expert witness offers access to the subject's truth from outside the specific discursive context of the trial. His knowledge of other subjects which can be said to form a set of subjects with similar psychological or behavioural traits allows him to speak the truth of the subject himself. For Foucault, the expert witness functions as 'the subject supposed to know'.[28] And in using this specific phrase, an echo of Lacan's definition of the transference in *Seminar XI*, Foucault invites us to think through the double role of psychoanalysis in analysis of legal proceedings and to consider this core psychoanalytic concept which appears to be operating on both sides of the law.

In order to elucidate this double play of psychoanalysis, it will be useful to investigate the specific function of psychiatric testimony in criminal trials. According to Foucault:

> [E]xpert psychiatric opinion allows the offense, as defined by the law, to be doubled with a whole series of other things that are not the offense itself but a series of forms of conduct, of ways of being that are, of course, presented in the discourse of the psychiatric expert as the cause, origin, motivation, and starting point of the offense. In fact, in the reality of judicial practice they constitute the substance, the very material to be punished.[29]

The testimony produces a certain truth of the subject that moves beyond the specific offense of which they are accused. Psychiatric testimony creates an origin for the subject that makes the offence only a symptom of their supposed innate predilections towards these forms of behaviour that are coded as transgressive. In doing so, the discourse of psychiatry eliminates doubt from the interpretations of the events by providing a clear trajectory from cause to event; in other words, it produces a meaningful narrative by which the subject's truth and, by extension, the truth of the forbidden act can be understood. The legal subject can then be understood and judged according to a standard of normality set by psychiatric discourse rather than the specific details of the case: the legal subject ceases to function as the sum of evidence proffered against her, but is now the construct of an exterior discourse that constructs for her an offence for which she is always already guilty. It is in this sense, then, that Foucault locates another doubling, that of the psychiatrist himself who functions as both witness and judge; a person who both constructs the nature of the subject and then proceeds to pass judgement on him.

There is a fundamental split, here, within my use of psychoanalysis as the discourse that questions all origins and destabilizes the hegemony of the proper name, and the instances of psychoanalytic discourse that Foucault discerns as fixing meaning and providing a discernible truth for the subject. It is important, here, not to be forced into the easy conclusion that these analysts did not understand Freud's message, that in these expert testimonies, we just are dealing with a grossly distorted reading of psychoanalytic material. This may well be the case, but it is imperative to trace this tension between, on the one hand, a transgressive discourse that questions all institutional claims to absolute truth, and on the other hand, a discourse that proceeds to name the ways in which this process takes place, thereby staking a claim to mastery over the process of naming thereby reproducing the role of the father that it wishes to kill.

This double figure of the analyst/judge emerges in Freud's *Introductory Lectures* of 1916. Freud here positions the discourse as fundamentally other to scientific or empirical discourses. First, Freud describes the discourses of medicine and psychiatry as based on what the practitioners 'see', linking the discourses to empirically based notions of truth.[30] He then describes the teacher of these discourses as 'a leader and interpreter who accompanies you through a museum, while you gain a direct contact with the objects exhibited and feel yourself convinced of the existence of the new facts through your own perception'.[31] The description of the teacher as a 'leader and interpreter', rather than a more benign or neutral phrase, emphasizes the degree to which the role of the teacher within this scenario is imbued with institutionally legitimated power, specifically the power to name the phenomena being perceived, and therefore influence the perceiving subject's interpretation of the 'facts' being perceived: this is the role of the judge and master. Already, in his depiction of empirical science, Freud is refocusing attention away from the subject of enunciation, the content of the teacher's speech, towards the enunciating subject, the presence of the speaker's desire. By doing so, Freud introduces the possibility of specific power relations involved in any declaration of truth as well as the presence of desire in the production of truth.

Freud then positions psychoanalysis as running counter to the means by which medicine and psychiatry asses the truth:

> In psychoanalysis alas, everything is different. Nothing takes place in psychoanalytic treatment but an interchange of words between the patient and the analyst. The patient talks, tells of his past experiences and present impressions, complains, confesses to his wishes and his emotional impulses. The doctor listens, tries to direct the patient's processes of thought, exhorts, forces his attention in certain directions and observes the reactions of understanding or rejection which he in this way provokes in him.[32]

Everything is different in psychoanalysis because it is especially tuned to the agency of the signifier in intersubjective relations. By implying that 'nothing takes place' except an exchange of words between two people, Freud surreptitiously implies that empirical science, too, is dependent upon the signifier. It is also important to note the different form that knowledge takes in Freud's description. The power of the doctor has to some degree lessened: instead of the 'leader' who tells the subject how to interpret, the psychoanalyst 'listens'. Whereas the medical doctor functions as a guardian to a privileged site of truth, the psychoanalyst takes a less assertive and collaborative approach with the patient. It is the patient who initiates the collaboration by speaking, and it is only in relation to the patient's words that the psychoanalyst is able to discern the subject's truth. The truth, here, is not the imagined stable and manageable one of empirical science; however, the analyst is only able to try and direct the route of the patient's discourse and his attempts are met with either understanding or rejection by the patient. The truth in psychoanalytic discourse is, then, always contingent upon words, which at any time could shift to a wholly new discourse, thus complicating, or shifting completely, the analyst's interpretation. We see, then, that psychoanalysis's emphasis on the agency of the signifier in the production of truth, a truth built upon a constantly shifting ground, is radically different from the empirical form of truth demanded by legal discourse.

Freud, later in the lecture series, returns to the figure of the analyst/judge in relation to the use of parapraxis as evidence for unconscious desires. He states that an analyst must always work with 'circumstantial evidence' and in doing so reintroduces the discourse of the law into psychoanalytic practice.[33] Imagining the audience's criticism of his interpretive methods, he ventriloquizes an imagined interlocutor, who voices similar concerns to Foucault's: 'Are you a judge, then? And is a person who has made a slip of the tongue brought up before you on a charge? So making a slip of the tongue is an offence, is it?'.[1] Rather than reject the comparison or accede to it, Freud, having introduced into the realm of knowledge a fundamental uncertainty, provides a more nuanced comparison of the two roles than given earlier:

> In the law courts it may be necessary for practical purposes to find a defendant guilty on circumstantial evidence. *We are under no such necessity*; but neither are we obliged to disregard the circumstantial evidence. It would be a mistake to suppose that a science consists entirely of strictly proved theses, and it would be unjust to require this. *Only a disposition with a passion for authority will raise such a demand, someone with a craving to replace his religious catechism by another, though it is a scientific one.* [...] It is actually a sign of a scientific mode of thought to find satisfaction in these approximations to certainty and to be able to pursue constructive work further in spite of the absence of final confirmation.[34]

The comparison between the law and psychoanalysis lies in their concomitant desire to discern the truth of the subject. However, Freud clearly delineates two very different desires at work here. The law demands a final answer out of 'necessity' and, as such, is forced to take circumstantial evidence as a stable ground upon which to decide. Psychoanalysis can allow for a much more unstable conception of the truth because its evidence is always circumstantial, it is always contingent upon the interaction between two or more subjects at any given time.

Psychoanalysis, unlike the law, functions on 'the absence of a final confirmation'. Any attempt to stop the process, to definitively name the truth of the subject, is symptomatic not of the truth being named but a desire on the part of the interpreter for 'authority'. The analyst with 'a passion for authority' who demands certainty from the psychoanalytic process is retranslating the process back into the discourse of the law. But what Freud sees as operative in that translation is a desire, not just for truth, but for power: here, we see Freud reaching the Nietzschean conclusion that the will to truth is but another manifestation of the will to power.

This relationship between desire and truth can be pursued further with recourse to Lacan's definition of the transference in *Seminar XI*. According to Lacan, the transference is the process by which 'the subject is looking for his certainty', a certainty denied to the subject by the constitutive deferral of meaning offered by the signifier.[35] The subject then seeks this missing wholeness in the Other, a 'subject supposed to know'.[36] The Other is imagined to have access to a truth denied to the subject and thus the subject demands from the Other the revelation of her consistency. This relation, however, belongs to the realm of fantasy whereby the subject's relation to her object of desire, her truth, is mediated through a fantasmatic screen, through which the Other with access to knowledge of this truth can be created. The subject accesses *jouissance* via the transference because her desire for knowledge of her consistency is always deferred and returned to. The knowledge that the subjects seeks in the Other is always unknown to him. It must remain unknown in order to maintain the fantasy and satisfy the drive.

The truth status of the knowledge in the transference is thus brought into question by the desire of the subject who desires, like Kafka's Ulysses, both knowledge and ignorance. Both Freud and Lacan suggest that the traversal of the transference is one of the first aims of a successful interpretation. If the analyst at any time performs the role of 'the subject supposed to know', he impedes the traversal of this fantasy. This is so because at any time the analyst is sure of the subject's truth, there is always the risk that he is acceding to the analysand's desire. This constitutes a failed analysis because the transference is a form of defence. As Lacan argues, 'far from being the handing over of powers to the unconscious, the transference is, on the contrary, its closing up'.[37] The analysand's relation to her own desire cannot be modified if the analyst, by performing the role of means to this desire's fulfilment, sustains the fantasy that requires traversal. To perform this role is to accede to the role of the 'unjust' judge with a fantasmatic 'craving' for certainty that Freud alludes to in his lecture.

The fantasy at play within the dynamic of the transference is belief in an exterior organizing principle around which the subject can organize her enjoyment. It is then a faith in the existence of a law impervious to the split between the subject of the enunciation and the enunciating subject. The suturing of the gap between the Symbolic and the Real through Imaginary identification with an unknown knowledge that the transference enacts is only possible through what Slavoj Žižek defines in *The Plague of Fantasies* as a fetishistic fixation:

> What characterizes human existence is [an] 'irrational' fixation on some symbolic Cause, materialized in a Master-Signifier to whom we stick regardless of the consequences, disregarding our most elementary interest, survival itself: it is the very 'stubborn attachment' to some Master-Signifier (ultimately a 'signifier without a signified') which enables man to maintain free flexibility towards every signified content.[38]

This Master-Signifier codes all other empty signifiers bestowing meaning and facilitating enjoyment in meaning. The link between this Master-Signifier and the other signifiers is not natural or stable; however, it is always contingent and political. As Žižek explains, '[t]he ideological struggle is precisely the struggle to impose an ever new meaning on this [empty signifier]'.[39] In order for the Master-Signifier to remain in its privileged place, the interpretation of it must be policed, and its truth must be routinely performed so as to appear natural. But it is at the moment of its re-suturing, when difference is silenced, that the contingency of the Big Other emerges most visibly: the same process occurs in legal discourse, the legal decision taken in the name of justice and natural right attests to the absence of justice at the same time as it violently rearticulates it.

The emergence of a Master-Signifier is itself a substitute for a constitutive gap between the Symbolic and the Real. It is in this logic of substitution that we can deduce within 'normal' sexuality the logic of fetishism. In *Three Essays on Sexuality*, Freud defines the fetishist as a subject for whom 'the normal sexual object is replaced by another which bears some relation to it, but is entirely unsuited to serve the normal sexual aim'.[40] The fetishistic structure involves a logic of substitution, an apparent divergence from a 'normal' sexual aim. But it is important to note that Freud's use of 'normal' is not moral or prescriptive but, rather, descriptive. In the *Introductory Lectures*, Freud locates numerous pathological and fetishistic structures within the field of 'normal' sexuality:

> Some perverse trait or other is seldom absent from the sexual life of normal people. Even a kiss can claim to be described as a perverse act, since it consists in the bringing together of two oral erotogenic zones instead of the two genitals. Yet no one rejects it as perverse; on the contrary, it is permitted in theatrical performances as a softened hint at the sexual act.[41]

The mouth of the lover in Freud's example is taken by the subject as a source of sexual pleasure, and it is a substitute for the 'normal' genital sexual act. In order to not be considered perverse, the mouth must not be perceived to be the sexual aim itself but, rather, be implied in a signifying chain that would lead to the sexual act. We have here the two definitions of the supplement: the kiss is both a replacement for the sexual act, in which case it is perverse, but also an addition to it and a guarantee of its meaning, and therefore normative. When the kiss signifies another signifier, that of the sexual relation, it is deemed normative. But when the signifying chain halts and the kiss signifies only itself, it is deemed perverse.

The act of kissing can then function as both perverse and normative depending on how it is enjoyed by the subject engaged in the act.

This split in the perception of the object is furthered by the potential for not only pleasure but also disgust. In the first of the *Three Essays*, Freud postulates that:

> a man who kisses a pretty girl's lips passionately, may perhaps be disgusted at the idea of using her toothbrush, though there are no grounds for supposing that his own oral cavity, for which he feels no disgust, is any cleaner than the girl's.[42]

The girl's mouth in this scenario functions both as the object of the man's desire and disgust. Nothing about the object has changed. An object can frequently function as a site of perverse enjoyment and phobic disgust not only for different subjects but also in the same subject. As such, the truth of the object, its proper place, finds its certainty neither in its own being nor in the subject who perceives it. It is the Master Signifier that sutures this gap and bestows upon the empty signifier of the mouth its meaning. But, as Freud insinuates, in the functioning of the Master-Signifier, there is also something perverse, a constant act of deferral from one signifier to another that can never reveal what it promises to name, in this case 'a normal sexual object'.[43] Žižek thus argues that this 'displacement is original and constitutive' because both relations to the signifier allow a fetishistic disavowal of castration.[44] Perhaps, then, the stages of psychosexual development named by Freud that go into making the normal adult can be interpreted as so many fetishistic substitutions for the lost and 'indefinite' polymorphous perversity of the child.[45] It is the given ideological field, with its incumbent Master-Signifiers that determine the type of enjoyment that the subject cultivates in relation to the Symbolic and, concurrently, what can be perceived as true.

The critic/judge

The fetishistic fixation upon Master-Signifiers and the means by which these structures are maintained can also be discerned in the history of literary criticism. In 'The Rise of English', Terry Eagleton traces a genealogy of literary criticism that begins in the mid-19th century that can supplement the failing discourses of religious truth: 'As religion progressively ceases to provide the social "cement", affective values, and basic mythologies by which a socially turbulent class-society can be welded together, "English" is constructed as a subject to carry this ideological burden from the Victorian period onwards'.[46] The study of English Literature in Britain emerges in a process of substitution, and the ideological field must depend upon the work of scholars to re-code the empty signifiers of the Symbolic with specific content that behoves the class interests of the bourgeoisie. We have then a failure of the transference: an ordering principle, God, is perceived to be impotent, and as such, literature is called upon as a substitute for the same aim, thus eliding the fact of castration and restoring consistency to the Symbolic. The discipline of English and the values it purports to be the truth of the literary object are part of a wider strategy to restore the fantasmatic screen between the law and the subject.

The key figure in this turn, according to Eagleton, is Matthew Arnold. Matthew Arnold defined the aim of criticism as an 'endeavour, in all branches of knowledge, theology, philosophy, history, art, science, to see the object as in itself it really is'.[47] In aligning the analysis of texts with the empirical sciences, Arnold subscribes to the empirical binary of truth/untruth and also a belief that the object of study can be perceived from a neutral perspective. What allows Arnold the freedom to interpret the objects of different cultures and domesticate their otherness is a fetishistic fixation upon the Master-Signifier 'Culture'. Arnold in *Culture and Anarchy* variously defines culture as 'sweetness and light', 'the disinterested endeavour after man's perfection' and the 'prevailing of the will of God'.[48] In all these definitions, no clear sense of what culture is emerges. Whenever Arnold attempts to show how these definitions work together, a certain tautological structure begins to emerge whereby each definition relies on being deferred onto another:

> The pursuit of perfection, then, is the pursuit of sweetness and light. He who works for sweetness works in the end for light also; he who works for light works in the end for sweetness also. But he who works for sweetness and light united, works to make reason and the will of God prevail.[49]

For Arnold, culture is made up of 'sweetness' and 'light'. A distinction is built between 'sweetness' and 'light' that, when brought together, constitute the achievement of 'perfection'. The achievement of perfection is concomitant with the making of 'reason' which is also synonymous with 'the Will of God'. The relation between sweetness and light is comparable to the relation between the signifier and the signified, in that the unification of both allows for a fixed meaning to emerge and thus reason in the way of cogent sense. That which sutures the gap between signifier and signified is the fantasy of the transference, the presence of a God that can guarantee a universal correspondence between words and material things. But, in order for this form of order to emerge, a fixation upon the Master-Signifier 'Culture', made up of sweetness and light, has to be in place: one that does not interrogate its structural necessity in the maintenance of this order. We have on the one hand the elucidation of the system that begins with the will of god and finds in sweetness and light their examples. However, we have on the other hand, and the very logic of the passage betrays this counter reading, the will of God being contingent upon two empty signifiers, which are in turn coded by the enigmatic signifier 'culture'. If we keep in mind Eagleton's diagnosis of the failing power of religious rhetoric, we can discern the process of a shift from the previous Master-Signifier of God onto its supplement and substitute, Culture.[50]

There is also present here, an edict that the task of the critic is to reveal the truth, to unveil mystifications and provide the reader with a previously hidden truth. Arnold is positioning himself and all critics who wish to follow his edicts as a subject supposed to know, to know the Will of God no less. This aspect of the transference as defined by psychoanalysis can be seen in Arnold's subsequent explanation of the desire of the critic:

> [the critic] obeys an instinct prompting [him] to try to know the best that is known and thought in the world, irrespectively of practice, politics, and everything of the kind; and to value knowledge and thought as they approach this best, without the intrusion of any other considerations whatever.[51]

The 'instinct' that Arnold describes would appear to be defined not only as an ethical and natural instinct but also a neutral one that is capable of disregarding politics. But it is under threat from possible intrusions of politics or the desire of the Other. The practice of the critic in the acquisition of knowledge is always under threat from the presence of the Other. And the act of criticism, the task of revealing knowledge, is then figured as a defensive formation against those forces which threaten the critic's capacity to know. And it is this capacity to know that brings with it enjoyment. Arnold's formulation not only denies the presence of the Other's desire but also the critic's own. Translating Arnold's 'instinct' into the drive of psychoanalysis, it can be perceived that despite the espousal of the absence of the critic's desire, the process that Arnold defines is the means by which the critic's desire is maintained. The neutral and knowable truth which criticism aspires to name cannot be separated from criticism's own stated desire to find it. The literary critic is, then, caught in the same transferential structures that Freud and Lacan identify at play within the clinic: A fetishistic fixation upon a Master-Signifier allows the critic to bestow upon the empty signifier a fixed meaning, eliding the issue of his own desire and the ideological basis of that desire. The function of criticism is not then to unveil hidden meaning in the empty signifier, but to bestow upon it a reading conducive to an ideological field bound together by a series of Master-Signifiers, signifiers that are continually referred to but never fundamentally questioned, and in doing so reproduces the structural logic of the fetish.

It is important to note the political dimension of this critical misidentification: The function of criticism corresponds to the function of the police. In T.S. Eliot's summation, criticism 'must always profess an end in view, which, roughly speaking, appears to be the elucidation of works of art and the correction of taste'.[52] Eliot's conception of criticism, like Arnold's, professes a norm, which is also presented as a moral good. But, in his definition, there remains an anxiety that the signifier can always be interpreted incorrectly. This anxiety is most readily evident in Eliot's own critical writing. Eliot argues that 'interpretation… is only legitimate when it is not interpretation at all, but merely putting the reader in possession of facts which he would otherwise have missed'.[53] The critic is again tasked with revelation of objective truth veiled by the signifier. The anxiety surrounding this task emerges with the admission that other interpretations may corrupt rather than correct: 'Fact can never corrupt taste… the real corrupters are those who supply opinion or fancy'.[54] The truth, and the good taste that can determine it, is always under threat from corrupt readings. In employing the language of corruption, Eliot echoes the legislative discourse of obscenity that seeks to protect the vulnerable from corruption. The function of criticism begins to coincide with the law and the policing of dissident readings and subjectivities.

And much like the legal and moral discourses that it echoes, Eliot's epistemology is also dependent upon a fixation on the signifier 'Culture' that allows him the ability to discern fact from fancy. Eliot's fetishistic attachment is to 'Tradition'. 'Tradition', according to Eliot, 'involves all those habitual actions, habits and customs, from the most significant religious rite to our conventional way of greeting a stranger, which represent the blood kinship of 'the same people living in the same place'.[55] Eliot's definition corresponds to Eagleton's previous definition of ideology quoted above. In both definitions, we are presented with a structure that co-ordinates a given subject's desire in a certain historico-political context. What is at stake in both Eliot and Arnold's criticism is the continual reconstitution of these co-ordinates. As Lacan argues in regards to *Hamlet*, 'Desire… finds in the fantasy its reference, its substratum, its precise tuning in the imaginary register'.[56] Counter to Eliot's claim that true criticism is on the side of fact and corruption of truth occurs with the interference of fantasy, I wish to advocate that the grounds upon which facticity can be based require a minimum of fantasy in order to function as facts. The basis upon which Eliot can argue that the Tradition offers access to truth is explained in his thesis of 'the disassociation of sensibility' set forth in his essay 'The Metaphysical Poets'.[57] Eliot states that '[t]he poets of the seventeenth century… possessed a mechanism of sensibility which could devour any kind of experience…. In the seventeenth century a disassociation of sensibility set in, from which we have never recovered'.[58] According to this theory, there existed a point in history where a non-arbitrary link between the signifier and the signified was possible, and no suture was required to link them. In Eliot's words, there remained no distance between 'thought' and 'experience'.[59] Tradition names the means by which what is truly poetry always aspires to recover this lost unity, offering a 'vital language'.[60] As in Arnold, we can locate a retrospective fantasy of unity as the basis for facticity to emerge. The fantasy of this fall from a previous natural relation between signifier and signified, the fixation upon this event, allows access to an Imaginary wholeness and is thus what all 'true' poetry achieves, and all criticism that is true has the task of revealing to the reader. It is a discourse of mastery that declares itself normal, decries perversion, whilst all the while relying upon a fetishistic disavowal of its own desire.

It is in keeping with this mode of reading that much of Joycean criticism has stayed loyal.[61] But as we have seen, this mode of reading betrays an ideologically motivated form of policing concurrent with and echoing the language of the law, even if it pretends to transgress it. Such methods are not compatible with the fundamentally antagonistic basis of knowledge presented in psychoanalysis, that is, the presence of a constitutive substitution disallowing any objective criteria or origin separate from the presence of desire. The result is a history of criticism that, in repeating the discourse of correction and corruption, fails to locate the obscene quality of a text other than by confirming or denying its obscenity according to the law's definition. Criticism without psychoanalysis, that is without the knowledge of the presence of the transference and the minimal degree of fantasy operative in any claim towards facticity, is doomed to repeat the edicts of the law, even if it sets out to critique it.[62] As Jacqueline Rose argues in *Sexuality and the Field of Vision*, '[t]he unconscious is the only defence against a language frozen into pure, fixed, or institutionalized meaning, and what we call sexuality, in its capacity to unsettle the subject, is a break against the intolerable limits of common sense'.[63] It is this break that psychoanalysis can both perceive and prompt within the bond between the Symbolic and the Imaginary fantasy. If there is a distinction to be drawn between the discourses of the law and psychoanalysis, it is that the law attempts to maintain the fantasy of unity by denying the presence of the unconscious whilst psychoanalysis actively attempts to keep the fissure open to locate the operation of the Real within the ideological field.

As we have seen, both the law and the discourse of literary criticism have relied upon a fantasmatic fall, an imagined period before the fall, and thus before the law. This fantasy functions as a point from which the desire to correct this fall can begin, a desire which can never find the fulfilment it seeks because the fall is constitutive of the desire itself. The fantasy of a previously correct state is from the very beginning corrupted, and it is this corruption at very origin of correction that instigates the desire to correct it. This is the short circuit that produces the belief in a unifying principle, a reading of a text that corresponds to the facts, and at the same time produces an anxiety that such facts need to be protected from corruption. It is thus that a psychoanalytic reading can produce a different knowledge of obscenity in that it can remain aware of the ambivalence at play in any rhetoric of corruption and fall. Instead of a corrective reading of the text, either correcting the legal discourse that condemned *Ulysses*, or the literary criticism that has fought to redeem the text, I would like to offer an alternative, 'corructive', reading.[64] The term 'corructive' is borrowed from the 'Night Lessons' chapter of *Finnegans Wake*, and in it, the two words 'corrective' and 'corrupted' can be discerned. In bringing the two words together, Joyce positions 'corructive' as neither corrupt nor correct, but as both and neither. As the law pertains to the correct, and corruption to transgression, we perhaps have operative in this word the fantasy of a moment before difference has emerged, before the law, a prelapsarian word. But, at the same time, difference does emerge for us to distinguish the undecidability between the correct and the corrupt. We require knowledge of the two words before we can fantasize a moment when difference has not yet emerged between them. The word 'corruction' neither finds its proper place before or after the fall. It can only emerge at the exact moment of the fall, as difference emerges. Dan Bristow locates 'Joycean ontology' in the lapsarian moment itself: thus, rather than there having been a pre-existing unity (pre-existing our disunity) to which we should strive to return, or a sudden entrance into a place which is always already a disunity, in which any idea of a previous unity is a lie, Joyce is taking as his springboard *the moment of the fall itself*.[65]

Following Bristow, we can trace a parallel between a Joycean and a psychoanalytic ontology. The moment of corruction is the moment of the slip of the tongue, the lapse in memory and the presence of the uncanny: in Bristow's terms, 'it is the (contingent) generation in the Real of our symbolic-imaginary status'.[66] Both the Joycean text and psychoanalysis emphasize the contingent and the antagonistic as productive as well as destructive. A criticism of Joyce or indeed any text that claims to be influenced by psychoanalysis must also remain attentive to the undecidable and the unconscious. It is this productive capacity that the law cannot allow and as such must repress. The result is a constitutive fetishist disavowal operative within the law and any discourse which proclaims objective truth.

A psychoanalytic reading of a literary text, an analysand's discourse or a trial, pays attention not to an elusive underlying truth which must be extracted by the reader. Instead, a psychoanalytic reading must be attuned to the waste, the dissonance and the non-sense of the discourse it studies. Peter Buse details this reading practice as an attentiveness to the overlooked, the seemingly inconsequential elements of the text:

> A psychoanalytic reading does not set out to explicate what a text means to say, but what it does not. It does not look to disinter a text's thesis, but fastens on the inconsequential, the unimportant element, that nevertheless insists. It is an oblique reading, one that cuts diagonally, as Lacan puts it. At the same time, its extractions do not aim at the cream, but at the scum.[67]

By aiming at that which the discourse of the trial does not need or desires to be expunged from the record, psychoanalysis allows us to perceive the investments and desires operative within the discourse itself, beyond, under and behind, the discourse's stated truth claim. In short, the scum is evidence of what needs to be taken away in order for the discourse to function, and this thesis seeks to analyse these conditions of possibility for a truth claim concerning a literary text within a legal context and the necessary scum that surfaces as a result.

Lawrence v Joyce/Life vs Life

With the theoretical and historical underpinnings of the project in place, I now wish to justify, or perhaps excuse myself for, the choice of James Joyce and D.H. Lawrence as the two authors whose trials will be the focus of this project. In response to the deconstruction and subsequent reconstruction of the modernist canon in an effort to offer a more inclusive, and indeed, accurate account of literary modernism, much recent modernist scholarship has moved away from Joyce and Lawrence as masculine masters. It is also important to note how the production of the tradition of modernism that was produced in the middle and latter parts of the 20th century is in many ways incongruous with the law's understanding of the texts it chose to prosecute. Modernism, what it is, what it does and how it differs from previous or other contemporary modes of literary production is not a key concern for the courts: and, as I shall discuss in length in Chapter 4, it is precisely the anachronism of *Lady Chatterley's Lover* that allows it to be figured as a palliative for a contemporary culture figured as corrupted by sex. The courts and vigilance societies targeted no particular type of literary text, modernism was just as much a target censorship as naturalist novels, popular texts intended for larger audiences and much earlier texts such as Boccaccio's *Decameron*. In this sense, the law operated independently of the categories created by literary criticism, and this fact should be recognized in any approach to these trials.

Recent critical works, such as Rachel Potter's *Obscene Modernism,* have emphasized this linkage between obscenity and modernist literary production, , and how this relationship effected the specific aesthetic practices of modernist writers and the genesis of their texts By arguing for or against modernism's relation to obscenity, these works tend to assume that the legal category itself is a stable one when, as I aim to prove, the law's approach to obscenity vastly differs depending on the nation, wording of the statute and the text itself. Instead, this thesis will align itself in some regard with Erik Bachman's challenge to analyse the failures inherent in the policing and codifying of obscenity: in *Literary Obscenities*, Bachman states that a reading of obscenity law should remain attentive 'both to the recurrent failure of courts at this time to formulate adequate tests for obscenity and to the ultimate failure of fiction to be deemed proscribably obscene'.[68] Whether critics have argued for the success of the literary text over the law, or the success of the law to properly appreciate the text, what is missing from these analyses is an attention to the manner in which the text fails to speak its truth and the law fails to name either the text's truth or its own. This failure is productive of the fantasies operative in order to give the effect of truth and to give the foundations for the right of the law to decide. Leaving to other scholars the important clarification of the modernist project's and individual artists' relation to the discourse of the law, this thesis will concern itself with the trials themselves and the investments that appear therein, investments which the specific literary text calls forth into the discourse of the law.

Key to the narrative that this thesis will offer is the introduction of literary criticism as a discourse of truth that inoculates the literary text from accusations of obscenity. For this reason, the two authors chosen for this thesis are two authors who in a sense came to dominate the study of English language literature in England and America: James Joyce and D.H. Lawrence. This choice is not an attempt to reinstate their value in the face of, especially in Lawrence's case, declining critical interest. Instead, I wish to argue that the trials of these two author's present excellent ways to analyse the shifting status and value of the literary text before and after the intervention of literary criticism.

Furthermore, within the history of literary criticism, Joyce and Lawrence have usually been positioned as a binary choice. Sometimes aesthetic, other times moral. W.W. Robson points to this polarity between the two authors when he writes that:

> [t]heir word divides opinions. Some readers dislike both. Some admire one and reject the other. Very few seem to care for both equally. This is because of the nature of their work. Each seems to make a claim for his kind of art as the right kind.[69]

These claims to truth have been taken up by the respective champions of these authors. Within the history of literary criticism's championing or denigration of either Joyce or Lawrence, one term that has been used to ascribe value to either author is their fidelity to life.

Within an important strand of literary criticism, exemplified most exuberantly by F.R. Leavis and the scholars associated with him and the journal *Scrutiny*, the term life took on a moral value. Those authors who were deemed to be on the side of life were deemed to be exemplars of a particular moral outlook that celebrated traditional values of community, ritual and a supposedly healthy relation to the natural world: Key among these authors and the starting point for Leavisite criticism was Lawrence. But this understanding of Lawrence and his texts as a means of accessing an alternative and affirmative relation to the world, of Lawrence as the prophet of an emancipatory politics came after his death. As I discuss in both Chapters 1 and 4, contemporary responses to Lawrence read him as exemplifying a threat to life, championing a dangerous form of sexuality and embodying a destructive *jouissance* that necessitated censure.

Joyce too has often been depicted as an author dedicated to the replication of life. The inclusion of sexuality and scatology within even the early works prompted the term life to be used either to disparage his writing as excessive or in a manner which celebrated its inclusion as fidelity to the lived experience of the characters he was attempting to represent. This fidelity to truth will be analysed in relation to the second Joyce trial; there, I will argue that, by figuring the text as on the side of life and truth, the defence successfully manages to absolve the accusations of the text's obscenity. But this stands in marked contrast to some of Joyce's more hostile critics who framed Joyce's experimental use of language as a movement away from life, wherein life is understood to be the material towards which a text should be gesturing. Carl Jung perceived in *Ulysses* a fundamental absence of life: for Jung

> hopeless emptiness is the dominant note of the whole book. It not only begins and ends in nothingness, but it consists of nothing but nothingness.

> It is all infernally nugatory. If we regard the book from the side of technical artistry, it is a positively brilliant and hellish monster-birth.[70]

Here, Joyce's text is depicted as mutation or perversion of life, its technical brilliance comes at the price of an abandonment of life itself. The nothingness the text signifies paradoxically becomes an excessive quality, with this absence being felt as overproximity to this perverse presence of negativity. The book is 'nugatory', without value, but again, this absence is figured as a presence, as a child, a child however who signifies an abomination which associates both author and text with evil and death.

What brings about this feeling of disgust is Joyce's fidelity not to truth or life but rather towards the signifier. This attentiveness to the materiality and mutability of the signifier corrupts the fantasmatic relation to the signifier itself, the sense of the signifier's natural relation to the world, its performative magic. In a review of early portions of *Finnegans Wake*, Sean O'Faolain voices similar anxieties about Joyce's experimental use of language:

> It is not merely ahistoric—not merely the shadow of an animal that never was, the outline of a tree that never grew, for even then we might trace it to some basic reality distorted and confused—but it comes from nowhere, goes nowhere, is not part of life at all. It has one reality only—the reality of the round and round of children's scrawls in their first copybooks, zany circles of nothing.[71]

Joyce's apparent mastery over language leads him to take not the place of the mature patriarch but the figure of the child just coming to grips with language, a pre-linguistic phase before symbolic castration has taken place. Joyce's writing is here an embodiment of the death drive, forcing its way back to the past, repeating it and in doing so presents the possibility of a beyond that is also the site of a fundamental absence. How a literary text can become an embodiment of the death drive will be a key concern for the first two chapters of this thesis. How the same text can come to embody life for literary criticism and the law will be the dominant theme of Chapters 3 and 4. What is called into question is the very polarity of these categories, with the texts and authors that come to stand in for them oscillating between extremes of meaning.

We have then two authors who supposedly offer an understanding of life itself. But their opposition to each other, their status as a binary choice, brings into disrepute the conceptual stability of the term life as a means to assess a text's meaning. A text can just as easily be figured as an embodiment of obscene destructive enjoyment as it can be figured as a source of social values and health. The way this truth of the text is constructed in the law courts and in the classrooms of the university will be analysed throughout this thesis. Chapters 1 and 2 will investigate the antagonistic relationship between the literary criticism and the law and the subsequent figuring of the text by the law as an embodiment of the death drive. Chapters 3 and 4 will go on to investigate the manner in which the law courts and the classroom form an alliance and together present the literary text as a life-bearing force. This alliance will be based upon the strategic desexualization of the text, a process which will be necessary in order to fix the text's truth and empower both the law and the university's capacity to police the reading subject's enjoyment.

Notes

1 Michel Foucualt, *The History of Sexuality Volume I: The Will to Knowledge*, trans. Robert Hurley, (London: Random House, 1988), p. 141.
2 Ibid. p. 143.
3 Sigmund Freud, *Totem and Taboo*, trans. James Strachey, (London: Routledge, 2001), p. 160.
4 Ibid. p. 164.
5 Ibid. pp. 164–165.
6 Ibid. p. 166.
7 Ibid.
8 Ibid.
9 Eric L. Santner, *My Own Private Germany: Daniel Paul Schreber's Secret History of Modernity*, (Princeton, NJ: Princeton University Press, 1996), p. 5.
10 Ibid. p. 7.
11 Ibid. p. 16.
12 Carl Schmitt, *Political Theology: Four Chapters on the Concept of Sovereignty*, trans. George Schwab, (Chicago, IL: University of Chicago Press, 2005), p. 5. Schmitt too perceives, in a much more overtly political discourse, the absence and the necessity for the state of exception that remains unthinkable according to the values of democratic liberalism. But where Freud and Schmitt differ is in the capacity for the sovereign right to decide to be successfully embodied; in Freud's myth, the living sovereign is ultimately impotent; whereas, in Schmitt, he is required to be potent. Where these views intersect however is the analysis that, in order for a society to function, a sovereign power must be felt by the subject to be operative, it is through fantasy that this perception and identification with the sovereign takes place.
13 Freud, *Totem*, p. 167.
14 Franz Kafka, 'The Silence of the Sirens', in *The Complete Stories*, trans. Willa Muir and Edwin Muir, (New York: Schocken, 1981), p. 272. Maurice Blanchot notes that this privilege of Ulysses over his crew is based upon his right to enjoyment and his ability to forbear seduction and enjoy modestly, within the edicts of the law:

> the stubbornness and caution of Ulysses, the treachery by which he took pleasure in the spectacle of the Sirens without risking anything and without accepting the consequences; this cowardly, mediocre and tranquil pleasure, this moderate pleasure, [...] this happy and confident cowardice, rooted in a privilege which set him apart from the common condition, the others having no right to such elite happiness.
>
> (Maurice Blanchot, 'The Song of the Sirens', in *The Station Hill Blanchot Reader*, trans. Lydia Davis, ed. George Quasha, (Barrytown, NY: Station Hill, 1999)), p. 444

15 Ibid.
16 Ibid.
17 Jacques Lacan, 'Kant with Sade', in *Ecrits*, trans. Bruce Fink, (London: Norton, 1999), pp. 646–670, p. 660.
18 Renata Salecl, *(per)Versions of Love and Hate*, (London: Verso, 2000), p. 59.

19 Kafka, 'The Silence of the Sirens', p. 272.
20 Salecl, *(per)Versions of Love and Hate*, p. 62.
21 Ibid.
22 Ibid. p. 66.
23 The source of this narrative is a codicil, a legal document that amends an original will or legal document. Although beyond the remit of this thesis, it is important to note that, in Kafka, as well as in numerous other literary texts, the law does not act as the agent of order, but, rather as an agent of disequilibrium. The irony played with by Kafka is that the will to truth operative in the law gives testimony to its own absent foundations. The aim of this book is to explore the opposite side of this encounter between law and literature: When the two discourses intersect within the law's domain, it is literature that is cast in the role of antagonist to truth and significant intellectual, physical and libidinal work is required to figure the literary text on the side of truth by literature's legal defenders.
24 Freud himself is not innocent of this charge as will be shown below. His constant oscillation between the subversive potential of psychoanalysis on the one hand (psychoanalysis as the plague), and a sincere belief in psychoanalysis being of use in criminal trials (the analyst as judge) testifies to this fundamental ambivalence not only in Freud, but the unconscious upon which he based the discourse.
25 Jacques Lacan, *Seminar XI: The Four Fundamental Concepts of Psychoanalysis*, trans. Alan Sheridan, (London: Karnac, 2004), p. 133.
26 Ibid. p. 132.
27 Michel Foucault, *Abnormal: Lectures at the College de France 1974–1975*, trans. Graham Burchell, (London: Verso, 2003), p. 13.
28 Ibid. p. 14. Here, Foucault is directly referencing Lacan's formulation of the transference, intimating a potential link between their thinking and in co-opting Lacanian discourse into his own critique perhaps suggests that the Lacanian mode of psychoanalysis offers an alternative to the one he is critiquing.
29 Ibid. p. 15.
30 Sigmund Freud, *Introductory Lectures on Psychoanalysis*, trans. James Strachey, (London: Penguin, 1991), p. 40.
31 Ibid. p. 41.
32 Ibid.
33 Ibid. p. 73.
34 Ibid. p. 73, emphasis mine.
35 Lacan, *Seminar XI*, p. 129.
36 Ibid. p. 131.
37 Ibid. p. 130.
38 Slavoj Žižek, *The Plague of Fantasies*, (London: Verso, 2008), p. 133.
39 Ibid. p. 119.
40 Sigmund Freud, 'Three Essays on Sexuality', trans. James Strachey, in *The Penguin Freud Library, Vol 7: On Sexuality*, (London: Penguin, 1991), p. 64.
41 Freud, *Introductory Lectures*, p. 364.
42 Freud, 'Three Essays', p. 64.
43 Ibid. p. 45.
44 Žižek, *Fantasies*, p. 135.
45 Freud, *Introductory Lectures*, p. 362.
46 Terry Eagleton, 'The Rise of English', in *Literary Theory: An Introduction*, (London: Blackwell, 2008), p. 21.
47 Matthew Arnold, 'The Function of Criticism at the Present Time', in *Essays in Criticism*, (London: Macmillan, 1865), pp. 1–42, p. 1.
48 Matthew Arnold, *Culture and Anarchy*, (Oxford: Oxford University Press, 2009), p. 31.
49 Ibid. p. 52.

50 It should be noted that both systems of Master-Signifiers are functioning at the same time, but that Arnold's text lays the foundation for the eventual replacement of one ideological code by another. It is in Arnold however that this relation between two forms of transference, the religious and the cultural, is most readily shown to share the same structure and political project.
51 Arnold, 'Criticism', p. 6.
52 Thomas S. Eliot, 'The Function of Criticism', in *Selected Prose*, ed. John Hayward, (London: Penguin, 1965), p. 18.
53 Ibid. p. 19.
54 Ibid. p. 20.
55 Thomas S. Eliot, 'After Strange Gods', in *Selected Prose*, ed John Hayward, (London: Penguin, 1965), p. 20.
56 Jacques Lacan, 'Desire and the Interpretation of Desire in *Hamlet*', in *Literature and Psychoanalysis: The Question of Reading Otherwise*, ed. by Shoshana Felman, (Baltimore, MD: Johns Hopkins University Press, 1982), pp. 11–52, p. 14.
57 Thomas S. Eliot, 'The Metaphysical Poets', in *Selected Prose*, ed. John Hayward, (London: Penguin, 1965), p. 111.
58 Ibid. p. 111.
59 Ibid. p. 110.
60 Ibid. p. 108.
61 It could, of course, be argued that recent trends in textual scholarship such as the emergence of genetic criticism, historicism and archival research as dominant practices in literary criticism have provided alternative forms of criticism that are not discourses of mastery. However, in each branch of these forms of criticism, certain fetishistic attachments are readily apparent in their methodologies. The apparent switch of emphasis towards the production of texts does not diminish the fetishistic attachment to the literary object but enforces it. As Žižek notes, the switch from the object to its production constitutes an inherent transgression within the framework delineated above:

> far from destroying the 'fetishist' illusion, the insight into the production mechanism in fact even strengthens it, in so far as it renders palpable the gap between the bodily causes and their surface-effect... In short, the paradox of 'the making of...' is the same as that of a magician who discloses the trick without dissolving the mystery of the magical effect.
>
> (Žižek, *Fantasies*, pp. 129–130)

Emphasis on the production processes constitutes a disavowal of the textual effects of the literary object upon both reader and critic, allowing the critic to enjoy the effects of the text uncritically.
62 That is not to say that psychoanalytic criticism of Joyce's texts cannot fall foul of the closing up of the unconscious that the transference facilitates. Carl Jung in '"Ulysses": A Monologue' uses the text to provide a diagnosis of Joyce and subsequently his daughter Lucia, as 'schizophrenic' (Carl G. Jung, *The Spirit in Man, Art and Literature*, trans. Richard F.C. Hull, (Abingdon: Routledge Classics, 2003), pp. 130–155, p. 141.) Jean-Michel Rabatè posits Lucia Joyce as the intended reader of *Finnegans Wake* and, in doing so, posits Lucia as a subject supposed to know (Jean-Michel Rabatè, *James Joyce and the Politics of Egoism*, (Cambridge: Cambridge University Press, 2001), p. 23). The figure of Lucia Joyce functions as the site upon which the burden of knowledge is frequently laid within Joyce criticism. In doing so, much criticism has also replicated the discourse of the trial by basing their claims to truth upon a fantasized Young-Girl.
63 Jacqueline Rose, *Sexuality in the Field of Vision*, (London: Verso, 2005), p. 3.
64 James Joyce, *Finnegans Wake*, (London: Wordsworth Classics, 2009), p. 300.

65 Dan Bristow, *Joyce and Lacan: Reading, Writing, and Psychoanalysis*, (London: Routledge, 2016), p. 35.
66 Ibid. p. 46.
67 Peter Buse, 'On the Diagonal: Jacques Lacan's Reading Lists', in *Parallax*, Vol. 22, No. 4, pp. 481–499, p. 486.
68 Erik Bachman, *Literary Obscenity: US Case Law and Naturalism after Modernism*, (University Park: Pennsylvania State University Press, 2018), p. 7.
69 Quoted in *Modernists at Odds: Reconsidering Joyce and Lawrence*, ed. Matthew J. Kochis and Heather L. Lusty, (Miami: University of Florida Press, 2015), p. 14.
70 Carl Jung, 'On *Ulysses*', in *James Joyce: The Critical Heritage Volume 2, 1928–41*, (London: Taylor & Francis, 2005), p. 512.
71 Sean O'Faolain, 'The Cruelty and Beauty of Words', in *James Joyce: The Critical Heritage Volume 2, 1928–41*, p. 392.

Bibliography

Arnold, Matthew, *Culture and Anarchy*, (Oxford: Oxford University Press, 2009).

———, 'The Function of Criticism at the Present Time', in *Essays in Criticism*, (London: Macmillan, 1865), pp. 1–41.

Bachman, Erik, *Literary Obscenity: US Case Law and Naturalism after Modernism*, (University Park: Pennsylvania State University Press, 2018).

Blanchot, Maurice, 'The Song of the Sirens', in *The Station Hill Blanchot Reader*, trans. Lydia Davis and ed. George Quasha, (Barrytown, NY: Station Hill, 1999), pp. 443–450.

Bristow, Dan, *Joyce and Lacan: Reading, Writing, and Psychoanalysis*, (London: Routledge, 2016).

Buse, Peter, 'On the Diagonal: Jacques Lacan's Reading Lists', in *Parallax*, Vol. 22, No. 4, pp. 481–489.

Eagleton, Terry, 'The Rise of English', in *Literary Theory: An Introduction*, (London: Blackwell, 2008), pp. 15–46.

Eliot, Thomas S., 'After Strange Gods', in *Selected Prose*, ed. John Hayward, (London: Penguin, 1965), pp. 23–31.

———, 'The Function of Criticism', in *Selected Prose*, ed. John Hayward, (London: Penguin, 1965), pp. 13–17.

———, 'The Metaphysical Poets', in *Selected Prose*, ed. John Hayward, (London: Penguin, 1965), pp. 7–10.

Foucault, Michel, *Abnormal: Lectures at the College de France 1974–1975*, trans. Graham Burchell, (London: Verso, 2003).

———, *The History of Sexuality Volume I: The Will to Knowledge*, trans. Robert Hurley, (London: Random House, 1988).

Freud, Sigmund, *Introductory Lectures on Psychoanalysis*, trans. James Strachey, (London: Penguin, 1991), p. 40.

———, 'Three Essays on Sexuality', in *The Penguin Freud Library, Vol 7: On Sexuality*, trans. James Strachey, (London: Penguin, 1991), pp. 125–248.

———, *Totem and Taboo*, trans. James Strachey, (London: Routledge, 2001).

Joyce, James, *Finnegans Wake*, (London: Wordsworth Classics, 2009).

Jung, Carl, 'On *Ulysses*', in *James Joyce: The Critical Heritage Volume 2, 1928–41*, (London: Taylor & Francis, 2005), pp. 584–586.

———, *The Spirit in Man, Art and Literature*, trans. Richard F.C. Hull, (Abingdon: Routledge Classics, 2003).

Kafka, Franz, 'The Silence of the Sirens', in *The Complete Stories*, trans. Willa Muir and Edwin Muir, (New York: Schocken, 1981), p. 272.

Kochis, Matthew J. and Heather L. Lusty (ed.), *Modernists at Odds: Reconsidering Joyce and Lawrence*, (Miami: University of Florida Press, 2015).

Lacan, Jacques, 'Desire and the Interpretation of Desire in *Hamlet*', in *Literature and Psychoanalysis: The Question of Reading Otherwise*, ed. Shoshana Felman, (Baltimore, MD: Johns Hopkins University Press, 1982), pp. 11–52.

———, 'Kant with Sade', in *Ecrits*, trans. Bruce Fink, (London: Norton, 1999), pp. 645–671.

———, *Seminar XI: The Four Fundamental Concepts of Psychoanalysis*, trans. Alan Sheridan, (London: Karnac, 2004).

O'Faolain, Sean, 'The Cruelty and Beauty of Words', in *James Joyce: The Critical Heritage Volume 2, 1928–41*, (London: Taylor & Francis, 2005), pp. 391–392.

Rabatè, Jean-Michel, *James Joyce and the Politics of Egoism*, (Cambridge: Cambridge University Press, 2001).

Rose, Jacqueline, *Sexuality in the Field of Vision*, (London: Verso, 2005).

Salecl, Renata, *(per)Versions of Love and Hate*, (London: Verso, 2000).

Santner, Eric L., *My Own Private Germany: Daniel Paul Schreber's Secret History of Modernity*, (Princeton, NJ: Princeton University Press, 1996).

Schmitt, Carl, *Political Theology: Four Chapters on the Concept of Sovereignty*, trans. George Schwab, (Chicago, IL: University of Chicago Press, 2005).

Žižek, Slavoj, *The Plague of Fantasies*, (London: Verso, 2008).

PART 1

~~The~~ Woman

All the women are one woman

In the first two trials examined in this thesis, the criterion used for ascertaining a text's obscenity was the Hicklin Test. The test derives from the English case of *R v Hicklin* (1868), wherein the text in question was an anti-Catholic pamphlet authored by Henry Scott and entitled *The Confessional Unmasked: shewing the depravity of the Romish priesthood, the iniquity of the Confessional, and the questions put to females in confession.*[1] Copies of the pamphlet were originally ordered to be destroyed, but Scott appealed the decision to the court of Quarter Sessions. Recorder Benjamin Hicklin rescinded the order of destruction on the grounds that it was not Scott's intention to 'corrupt and deprave' the public, but rather to expose barbaric practices within the Catholic Church. A second appeal, this time by the prosecution and conducted at the Queen's Bench, revoked Hicklin's decision arguing that the intention of the author was irrelevant when deciding whether a publication was obscene. In his ruling, Chief Justice Alexander Cockburn set down what would become known as the Hicklin Test which would be used to justify the great majority of the subsequent prosecutions under the 1857 Obscene Publications Act in Britain and Under the Comstock Act in the United States.[2] Cockburn held that, in order for the prosecution to prove a text obscene, it must demonstrate a 'tendency… to deprave and corrupt those whose minds are open to such immoral influences, and into whose hands a publication of this sort may fall'.[3] Cockburn's decision to shift the determinate of guilt from the author onto the reader engendered a shift in the hermeneutic practices of all subsequent trials.

DOI: 10.4324/9781003202509-1

The Hicklin test is the first instance in this text of a persistent legal fantasy of a prelapsarian form of purity that is under threat from an obscene form of *jouissance*. Commenting on Scott's text, Cockburn emphasizes the degree to which this imagined pure subject is threatened by a destructive and seditious exterior agent:

> This work, I am told, is sold at the corners of streets, and in all directions, and of course it falls into the hands of persons of all classes, young and old, and the minds of those hitherto pure are exposed to the danger of contamination and pollution from the danger it contains.[4]

It is the law's duty to intervene in order to maintain the purity of this imagined vulnerable subject. The signifier itself comes under suspicion in this legal definition, its dissemination and interpretation cannot be contained, neither can the form of enjoyment it elicits be pre-determined.

It is also important to notice that the movement of emphasis from an author to a reader is also a movement from a known legal subject to an abstract and undefined reader. Within legal discourse, the author no longer operated as the locus onto which the meaning of a text can be fixed. Instead, the meaning and, consequently, the danger of a text could be determined by its effects on its reader. This reader, however, is not an ideal or average reader but a susceptible one who needs to be protected from the possibility of corruption.

The use of the specific terms 'deprave' and 'corrupt' in the discourse of the trials has important connotations for this study, also. To deprave, from the Latin *prāvus*, crooked implies a norm from which to gauge the perversion that a text could cause. It then becomes the task of the legal trial to agree upon a norm from which deviation can take place. To corrupt, meaning to spoil or destroy also implies the presence of a foreign agent who performs the corruption. The rhetoric of corruption, with its biological connotations, indicates the degree to which the law is not only interested in the policing of texts but also of living bodies, specifically women's: in this coinciding of the norm and the body, the biopolitical aspects of Hicklin become clear.

By figuring itself as the protector of this purity, the law can thus operate as pure itself and absolve itself of any of the enjoyment it perceives at play in the text. The positing of a vulnerable subject and the necessity to protect her thus allows the law to disavow its own status as writing, as a product of the very same structure of language that it treats with suspicion.

In both of the following trials, this imagined reader will be specifically figured as feminine and under threat from the literary texts on trial. In order to better understand this legal investment in the purity of female readers, I will briefly delineate the Lacanian understanding of ~~The~~ Woman as one of the instances of the Name-of-the-Father. By understanding how the law does not protect but actually produces this figure in order to justify its operation, I hope to show how this fantasy underpins both the trial of *The Rainbow* and *The Little Review*.

Lacan begins Seminar XX with a discussion of ontology. The history of ontology, both in philosophic and mythical forms, has routinely posited the sexual relationship as the ground for describing the essence of the cosmos. Lacan does not urge a return to these systems of thought but, rather, he asks why they always return to the sexual relationship in order to justify themselves. The ubiquity of these myths does not point to a universal truth. Instead, it attests to the universal 'failure of the sexual relationship' that this excess seeks to compensate for.[5] Love, and its attendant signifiers, functions as the means of eliding the sexual relationship rather than confirming it: 'they revolve', Lacan argues, 'around the fact that there's no such thing as the sexual relationship'.[6] The multitude of myths that use the sexual relationship attests to the degree to which the real of sexual difference, that traumatic kernel that resists symbolization, pervades the entirety of language, the failure at an individual level is deferred on to the family, on to the community, until the entire cosmos must stand as the justification for the sexual relationship. And it is not just in the obviously sexualized ontologies that this failure can be recognized: discussing Aristotle's *Nichomachean Ethics*, Lacan argues that, here too, we find the same deadlock. In his attempt to construct an ethics by which the world can be understood, Aristotle must assert certain universals (The Good, Truth, Beauty) that act as guarantors for the system of meaning. Lacan's point is that the need for these universals is necessitated by a certain constitutive lack in the system itself; that these universals need to be enunciated is evidence of the lack of their own self-evidence. The *jouissance* offered by the system fails, it requires an 'other satisfaction [...] that can be seen to emerge from [...] the universals: the Good, Truth, and Beauty'.[7] In the overtly sexuated cosmology of myth or in any secular ethics, 'something skids off track in what is manifestly aimed at, and then it immediately starts up with the good and happiness'.[8]

There would seem to be no escape from this deadlock. 'Reality', Lacan claims, 'is approached with apparatuses of *jouissance*' and 'there's no other apparatus than language. That is how *jouissance* is fitted out in speaking beings'.[9] Language thus operates as the medium by which the subject accesses *jouissance*, and it is *jouissance* that mediates reality. However, Lacan insists that this fact does not indicate 'that *jouissance* is prior to reality'; *jouissance* is only possible once a signifying system is in place to designate its movement.[10] Any signifying system that attempts to totalize the world under the auspices of the signifier must, like Aristotle's ethics, miss the mark, come short in some way. This failure is a productive one in that it introduces a circuit that can be infinitely repeated by the drive. This *jouissance* that fails and is doomed to repeat is phallic *jouissance*, and Lacan will designate it structurally as male. There is also (an)Other *jouissance* that Lacan designates as female. This *jouissance* is predicated on the existence of the exception to the signifying system, 'on the basis of the not whole'.[11] The feminine position of 'not all' points to the radical contingency of the law, the degree to which the signifier bears no natural relationship to the signified or the world it hopes to represent. The existence of the feminine position of not all potentially indicates the possibility that these symbolic fictions can be rewritten that the co-ordinates of the subject's desire can be reformulated.

For Lacan, male and female constitute two structural positions within language. The two positions do not necessarily coincide with a given subject's biological sex or a culturally designated gender but rather with the subject's relation to language and the concomitant modes of *jouissance* available to her. Slavoj Žižek succinctly glosses the distinction when he states that:

> sexual difference does not designate any biological opposition grounded in "real" properties but a purely symbolic opposition to which nothing corresponds in the designated objects—nothing but the Real of some undefined *x* that cannot ever be captured by the image of the signified.[12]

In *Seminar XX*, Lacan details this logic of sexuation. The male relationship to language and the form of *jouissance* available to him is centred around the phallus, not understood as the biological penis, although, in some sense, the penis can function as its proxy, but rather as the structuring principle of the male's relationship to the symbolic and imaginary, in a word, fantasy. The phallus in Lacanian psychoanalysis is a structuring principle through which the male subject learns to desire and finds his position in relation to the Other, as its lover. Following this logic, then, for the male, there is only one form of *jouissance*, all *jouissance* is phallic *jouissance*.

But there exists a fundamental gap between the male subject's desires and their articulation into signifiers, so much so that these desires are never fully satiated. The phallus, in all its symbolic weight, functions not only as a fantasy of the male subject's potency and identity but also as the means overcoming this symbolic castration by the signifier. This dynamic produces the *object petit a*, as a supplement to phallic *jouissance* that allows for a fantasmatic relation to the other, that allows him to be the other's lover. The *object a* is, according to Lacan,

> from at least one pole of sexual identification, the male pole - the object that puts itself in the place of what cannot be glimpsed of the Other. It is inasmuch as *object a* plays the role somewhere - from a point of departure, a single one, the male one - of that which takes the place of the missing partner, that what we are also used to seeing emerge in the place of the real, namely, fantasy, is constituted.[13]

The barred subject can only approach the feminine in the form of *object a*, the partial object and object cause of desire. According to Lacan, man may indeed 'believe he approaches woman', and in doing so attempts to achieve a harmonious sexual relationship, 'but what he approaches is the cause of his desire that I have designated as *object a*. That is the act of love'.[14] This act of love is destined to fail as it aims towards the partial object and not the female subject herself: 'He is unable to attain his sexual partner, who is the Other, except inasmuch as his partner is the cause of his desire'.[15] We have here a Lacanian reproduction of the myth of the sirens, wherein the male investment in a form of knowledge beyond the signifier is manifested in the fantasy of seduction by ~~The~~ Woman. However, this act of love not only threatens death but it also helps to maintain the symbolic life of the male subject; it maintains his desire. The male subject is caught in the perpetual work of maintaining the proper proximity to the object of desire. Lacan suggests the repetitive drive at work within the process of maintaining this fantasy when he states 'Man believes he creates – he believes believes believes, he creates creates creates. He creates creates creates woman. In reality, he puts her to work - to the work of the One'. Male desire is figured as narcistic, it creates ~~The~~ Woman to assist in the erasure of the lack within the phallus, the creation of the One. It is also figured as exploitative; ~~The~~ Woman is here being put to work for his enjoyment. But also, through the repetition of the acts of belief and creation also hints at the futility of these actions and the presence of the drive, maintaining itself through perpetual failure and return.

We have previously witnessed such an incarnation of full enjoyment in the figure of the primal father whose murder allows for the origin of the law. Salecl discusses this similarity between the fantasy figure of ~~The~~ Woman and the Primal father of Freud's myth when she notes that '[i]n the case of Woman—the mythical "She"- [...] we are dealing with an agency of power that is presymbolic, unbridled by the law of castration'.[16] In referring to ~~The~~ Woman as uncastrated, we can see a clear link between this fantasy figure and the full enjoyment of the primal father. But as a figure with whom the male subject can hope to conquer or possess, ~~The~~ Woman's function differs slightly from the primal father in that she remains very much alive as a fantasy and as such presents the possibility of access to a form of enjoyment beyond the castrating signifier.

The fantasized enjoyment of ~~The~~ Woman does not correspond to the enjoyment of a feminine subject in *Seminar XX*. After his discussion of the deadlock of phallic *jouissance*, the paradox of feminine *jouissance* is introduced. Lacan argues that there exists an exception to the law of the father, a *jouissance* that is not phallic; feminine *jouissance*. This is the exception that escapes any attempt to be signified.

Unlike the male whose enjoyment of the signifier is governed by the phallus, not all the female's *jouissance* is phallic. But because all *jouissance* that exists within language is phallic *jouissance*, and the phallus governs the relation of the subject to language, this Other enjoyment that the feminine subject has access to must exist outside language. This doesn't preclude her from phallic enjoyment, from enjoying 'like a man' but means she can enjoy in more than way, her relationship to the signifier is not one of complete subordination. The feminine subject, following this argument, perhaps has a choice as in what way she enjoys. According to Lacan, 'If [feminine *jouissance*] inscribes itself [in the Symbolic], it will not allow for any universality – it will be a not-whole, insofar as it has the choice of positing itself [...] or of not being there'.[17]

We have here two versions of ~~The~~ Woman: the fantasized object of desire produced by the male subject whose acquisition would return to him the wholeness lost during his admittance to the Symbolic. But also, a feminine version. This version of ~~The~~ Woman, a term Lacan chooses to bar as the exception to the phallic symbolic order, is defined by its being 'not whole' and cannot therefore be said to exist: this is why the definite article, 'La' is struck through in Lacan's graph: there is no stable universal Woman because her existence as 'not all' intimates not an exterior truth but an exterior impossibility, a failure of the Symbolic to name her whole truth. Cecilia Sjöholm clarifies the female subject's liminal relation to the Symbolic when she argues that:

> [t]here is not the woman in the universal sense, no feminine subjectivity that lends itself to the universalizability that language allows us to indicate. Femininity is not defined by the universal signifier of the woman, because there is no symbol that would supplement and define the signifier of woman with a possible notion of her desire, for instance.[18]

The failure of the symbolic to name and speak the woman's desire thus places her desire outside the symbolic and poses it as a question to the male subject perceiving it. Which, in turn, brings us back to the fantasy figure of ~~The~~ Woman. ~~The~~ Woman is a response to the absence perceived by the male in the female subject: ~~The~~ Woman is the male subject's answer to the question of the female subject's desire. But the existence of the female subject and the presence of an unspeakable enjoyment, an enjoyment that, because it is unspeakable is therefore an enjoyment in untruth, threatens the promise of uncastrated enjoyment that the male perceives in ~~The~~ Woman's seduction. In short, the female subject and her enjoyment put the male's enjoyment of his fantasy at risk.

In her book *Females*, Andrea Long Chu puts forward a simpler but no less radical proposition: 'Everyone is female, and everyone hates it'.[19] For Chu, being female constitutes:

> any psychic operation in which the self is sacrificed to make room for the desires of another. These desires may be real or imagined, concentrated or diffuse—a boyfriend's sexual needs, a set of cultural expectations, a literal pregnancy—but in all cases, the self is hollowed out, made into an incubator for an alien force. To be female is to let someone else do your desiring for you, at your own expense.

To be female, for Chu, is the default ontological position of the subject in so much as to be necessarily implicates the subject in the Other's desire. Our status as speaking-beings already presupposes the presence of the other: language is not our own, it is loaned from the Other, and the symbolic payment demanded by the other for this debt is castration. To come into language is, following Lacan and Chu, the becoming female of the subject.[20]

Chu's analysis helps us move further away from the potential for biological essentialism in both Freud and Lacan and helps us root sexual difference in a relation to both cultural demands and forms of enjoyment:

When I talk about females, I am not referring to biological sex, though I'm not referring to gender, either. I'm referring instead to something that might as well be sex, the way that reactionaries describe it (permanent, unchanging, etc.), but whose nature is ontological, not biological. Femaleness is not an anatomical or genetic characteristic of an organism, but rather a universal existential condition, the one and only structure of human consciousness. To be is to be female: the two are identical.[21]

Psychoanalysis's insistence on sexual difference and a process of sexuation instead of gender can thus be defended on Chu's terms. To exist is to inhabit the Symbolic, to incorporate the other's discourse, and as such, the other's desire into one's innermost core. The price of entry, as outlined above, is the presence of an alien force disqualifying any complete identity and disqualifying any sense of authenticity. This analysis allows for an understanding of both the male side of Lacan's graph and ~~The~~ Woman who maintains his access to *jouissance* as fantasmatic formations produced by a fundamental disavowal of the feminine. This analysis also allows us to include that not designated female at birth as both Chu and Lacan are more interested in positions taken in relation to an existential condition:

> Everyone is female, but how one *copes with* being female—the specific defense mechanisms that one consciously or unconsciously develops as a reaction formation *against* one's femaleness, within the terms of what is historically and socioculturally available—this is what we ordinarily call *gender.*[22]

Gendered identities are those made against the subject's original femaleness, a fantasy formation designed to shield the subject from its own inability to master the world. The variation and behaviours of these identities are not fixed but subject to the cultural, historical and technological contexts in which the subject can choose or are allocated a specific identity. But is important to stress that this identification, and any form of identity politics that emerges from these positions, is always itself a misidentification of a constitutive maladjustment within the Symbolic Order: however, you identify that identification is not your own and in order to do so requires a constitutive misidentification with the signifier. Instead of an identity politics, where we find what is in us more than ourselves within stable categories and behaviours, we inhabit a politics of identification, wherein the intersection of desire and the signifier trouble any sense of belonging within the Symbolic Order.

I do not intend this argument to be a reactionary call for an abolishment of contemporary identity politics in the sense of a return to a previous 'simpler' relation between sexes. To do so would be to make the naïve error that any previous political regime did not require an identification with a master–signifier of some sort be it whiteness, Christ, the sovereign or the nation state: *There is no politics that is not always already an identity politics.* But the important point to take away from Chu's analysis is the manner in which these forms of politics, however, inclusive and emancipatory they may seem, always necessitate an abjection of the feminine: 'The political is the sworn enemy of the female; politics begins, in every case, from the optimistic belief that *another sex is possible*'.[23] The female is excluded in so far as that which is excluded is always coded as feminine in this analysis.

The law, I wish to argue, is one apparatus through which politics shapes the fantasy of another sex: maleness is structured and maintained by the law in the form of the paternal metaphor or names-of-the-father but is itself a fantasy construct designed to offer refuge from the subject's primary femininity. Here, we find a variation on Alfred Adler's concept of masculine protest. In his 1910 paper, 'Inferiority Feeling and Masculine Protest', Adler posits that for both male and female children, an identification with the mother is rejected in favour of the father leading to a jettisoning of the feelings and behaviours identified with the mother. As Adler goes on to argue:

> Every form of inner compulsion in normal and neurotic individuals may be derived from this attempt at a masculine protest. Where it succeeds, it naturally strengthens the masculine tendencies enormously, posits for itself the highest and often unattainable goals, develops a craving for satisfaction and triumph, intensifies all abilities and egotistical drives, increases envy, avarice, and ambition, and brings about an inner restlessness which makes any external compulsion, lack of satisfaction, disparagement, and injury unbearable. Defiance, vengeance, and resentment are its steady accompaniments.[24]

For Adler, the process of masculine protest in males is a natural process which strengthens the subject and thus allows him to overcome his initial reliance upon the feminine other becoming an individual agent. Adler would later revise this concept and use the term only to refer to female subjects who refuse to identify with the cultural demands to perform the cultural demands of passivity and nurturing. However, for our analysis, this early account can be applied less so to individuals but expanded into a shared cultural and existential condition that gives rise to a form of transference, an identification with the law itself as the guarantor of the male subject's phallic *jouissance*.

Freud's theorization of Schreber's paranoia understands masculine protest as itself a paranoid response to latent or repressed homosexual desire. Commenting on Schreber's belief that he was being transformed into a woman so as to give birth to the offspring of a vengeful and sadistic God, another version of the primal father of pure *jouissance*, Freud argues that Schreber's incredibly complex fantasies amounting to an entire cosmology constitute a concerted attempt to disavow those homosexual desires. Paranoia and its incumbent fantasies of persecution, for Freud, are 'an attempt at recovery, a process of reconstruction'.[25] The paranoid fantasy allows Shreber access to an enjoyment he once had. For Freud, Schreber's paranoid fantasies allow for the dethatched libidinal cathexis for the father to assert themselves, thus allowing him to posit a definitive homosexual cause for paranoia.

Building on Freud's analysis whilst significantly expanding it, Santner posits that Schreber's God is not only a projection of his own sadistic father but also is directly linked to a realization concerning his profession: before the onset of his paranoia, Schreber had recently been promoted to Senatspräsident, a senior judge and an embodiment of the law itself. The return of the sadistic fantasies and identification as a woman is concomitant with a revelation concerning the law and his inability to embody it. According to Santner, Schreber's symptoms and his later memoirs constitute 'a form of knowledge concerning profound malfunctions in those politicotheological procedures that otherwise sustain the very ontological consistency of what we call the "world"'.[26] The co-ordinates of not only his desire but also the shared fantasies of the culture in which they inhabit, fantasies maintained by the law, come apart in light of the law's inconsistency, the lack of any objective grounding of its claims to truth. The obscene God of Schreber's delusion is the same obscenity he located in the law, and his feminization is an attempt to return to, in an inverted and perverse form, the sexual relation. The law itself, according to this understanding, is a paranoid construct designed to maintain a strict binary between The Phallus and The Woman, a fantasized sexual relation that obscures the subject's primary femininity.

To summarize: The first 'other sex' identity to be created is the male, which is then posited as primary so as to abject the repressed feminine aspect onto those 'select delegates' coded as women. In this sense, we could also further radicalize Lacan's graph by not only drawing a line through the definite article of Woman but also Phallus and posit the entire schema not as a source of truth about the essence of sexual difference but as an elaborate diagram of interlocking fantasies: the male side is itself a fantasy formation designed to disguise the primary femininity of the subject whose desire is co-ordinated by its inability to find the locus of its enjoyment within the confines of the Symbolic Order. This fantasy requires a supplement, a partner in crime, an object who if obtained could relieve the male of the discontent it finds with the signifier. This is Woman. The law's function, a fundamentally paranoid one, is to police and maintain this fragile and complex series of fantasies by attempting to protect this crucial supplement to phallic enjoyment.

With this dynamic in mind, the paranoid fantasmatic underpinnings of Hicklin become clearer: by conceiving of the vulnerable feminine reader as a site of purity and the text as the obscene corrupter, obscenity law functioned as a means of preserving the figure of Woman, protecting male enjoyment and figuring the work of feminine *jouissance* in the literary text. In the following two chapters, I will show how this fantasmatic investment in a universal woman and a related vulnerable reader in need of the law's intervention plays out in both the trials of *The Rainbow* and *The Little Review*. In *The Rainbow* trial, we shall witness the crisis of representation the figure of the lesbian produces in the law's ability to police the proper name: the lesbian comes to figure an obscene double to ~~The~~ Woman who offers no potential seduction to the male subject and threatens to seduce ~~The~~ Woman herself, thus robbing the male subject of the truth and enjoyment she offers.

Notes

1 Wayne C. Bartee and Alice F. Bartee, *Litigating Morality: American Legal Thought and Its English Roots*, (New York: Praeger, 1992), p. 85.

2 The Act did not, however, define obscenity. It was not until *R v Hicklin* that any working definition was applied. The Hicklin test became the test of obscenity until the Act's repeal in 1957.

Prosecutions under the Act included Henry Vizetelly, the publisher of English translations of Emile Zola's novels (1888), D.H. Lawrence's *The Rainbow* (1915), James Joyce's *Ulysses* (1922), Radclyffe Hall's *The Well of Loneliness* (1928), Lawrence's *Lady Chatterley's Lover* (1929) and Henry Miller's *Tropic of Cancer* (1934).

3 Quoted in Bartee and Bartee, *Litigating Morality*, p. 85.

4 Quoted in Minette Hillyer, 'Sex in the Suburban: Porn, Home Movies, and the Live Action Performance of Love in Pam and Tommy Lee: Hardcore and Uncensored', in *Porn Studies*, ed. Linda Williams, (London: Duke University Press, 2004), pp. 33–75, p. 74.

5 Jacques Lacan, *Seminar XX: On Feminine Sexuality, The Limits of Love and Knowledge*, trans. Bruce Fink, (London: Norton, 1999), p. 18.

6 Ibid. p. 57.

7 Ibid. p. 53.

8 Ibid. p. 55.

9 Ibid.

10 Ibid. p. 54.

11 Ibid. p. 72.

12 Slavoj Žižek, 'The Real of Sexual Difference', in *Reading Seminar XX: Lacan's Major Work on Love, Knowledge, and Feminine Sexuality*, ed. Bruce Fink and Suzanne Barnard, (Albany: SUNY Press, 2002), pp. 42–80, p. 47.

13 Lacan, *Seminar XX*, p. 63.

14 Ibid. p. 56.

15 Ibid. p. 72.

16 Renata Salecl, *Sexuation*, (London: Duke University Press, 2000), p. 9.

17 Ibid. p. 80.

18 Cecilia Sjöholm, *The Antigone Complex: Ethics and the Invention of Feminine Desire*, (Stanford, CA: Stanford University Press, 2004), p. 95.

19 Andrea L. Chu, *Females*, (London: Verso, 2019), p. 13.

20 This does beg the question of what comes before the entry into language: is the child not sexed before the intervention of the signifier? It is beyond the scope of my current investigation, but we can look to Melanie Klein's work of the pre-oedipal ambivalence towards the originary object of the mother's breast and a universal primary femininity that must be disavowed by the male child to look for further causes and explanations of Chung's claims.

21 Ibid. p. 13.

22 Ibid. p. 14.

23 Ibid.

24 Alfred Adler, 'Inferiority Feelings and Masculine Protest', in *The Individual Psychology of Alfred Adler: A Systematic Presentation in Selections from His Writings*, ed. Heinz L. Ansbacher and Rowena R. Ansbacher, (New York: Basic Books, 1956), pp. 45–52, p. 46.

25 Sigmund Freud, 'Psychoanalytic Notes on an Autobiographical Account of a Case of Paranoia', in The *Standard Edition of The Complete Psychological Works of Sigmund, Freud: Volume XII*, ed. and trans. James Strachey, (London: Hogarth Press, 1981), p. 71.

26 Eric L. Santner, *My Own Private Germany: Daniel Paul Schreber's Secret History of Modernity*, (Princeton, NJ: Princeton University Press, 1996), p. xiii.

Bibliography

Adler, Alfred, 'Inferiority Feelings and Masculine Protest', in *The Individual Psychology of Alfred Adler: A Systematic Presentation in Selections from His Writings*, ed. Heinz L. Ansbacher and Rowena R. Ansbacher, (New York: Basic Books, 1956), pp. 45–52.

Bartee, Wayne C. and Alice F. Bartee, *Litigating Morality: American Legal Thought and Its English Roots*, (New York: Praeger, 1992).

Chu, Andrea L., *Females*, (London: Verso, 2019).

Fink, Bruce, 'Knowledge and Jouissance', in *Reading Seminar XX: Lacan's Major Work on Love, Knowledge, and Feminine Sexuality*, ed. Bruce Fink and Suzanne Barnard, (Albany: SUNY Press, 2002), pp. 21–46.

Freud, Sigmund, 'Psychoanalytic Notes on an Autobiographical Account of a Case of Paranoia', in The *Standard Edition of The Complete Psychological Works of Sigmund, Freud: Volume* XII, ed. and trans. James Strachey, (London: Hogarth Press, 1981), pp. 9–85.

Hillyer, Minette, 'Sex in the Suburban: Porn, Home Movies, and the Live Action Performance of Love in Pam and Tommy Lee: Hardcore and Uncensored', in *Porn Studies*, ed. Linda Williams, (London: Duke University Press, 2004), pp. 33–75.

Lacan, Jacques, *Seminar XX: On Feminine Sexuality, The Limits of Love and Knowledge*, trans. Bruce Fink, (London: Norton, 1999).

Salecl, Renata, *Sexuation*, (London: Duke University Press, 2000).

Santner, Eric L., *My Own Private Germany: Daniel Paul Schreber's Secret History of Modernity*, (Princeton, NJ: Princeton University Press, 1996).

Sjöholm, Cecilia, *The Antigone Complex: Ethics and the Invention of Feminine Desire*, (Stanford, CA: Stanford University Press, 2004).

Žižek, Slavoj, 'The Real of Sexual Difference', in *Reading Seminar XX: Lacan's Major Work on Love, Knowledge, and Feminine Sexuality*, ed. Bruce Fink and Suzanne Barnard, (Albany: SUNY Press, 2002), pp. 42–80.

1

METHUEN V METHUEN

D.H. Lawrence's novel *The Rainbow* was published on 30 September 1915. Two months later, the text was charged under the 1856 Obscene Publications Act. Lawrence was not legally accountable for his text; instead, the publisher Methuen was liable for printing the novel. The hearing was held at Bow Street Magistrates Court in London. Beyond the newspaper reports of the proceedings, the sole legal trace of the trial is to be found in the court ledger held in The City of London Archive. Betwixt two cases of offences against the Trading with the Enemy Act 1914, and a case of impersonating an officer of the British Army, a single line denotes the name of Methuen, the offence of obscene publication, the guilty verdict and the financial penalty accrued. The quotidian nature of the recording of the trial stands in stark contrast to the series of escalating media spectacles that will constitute the future trials. The legal context of the trial also places the prosecution of the literary text within the larger context of the ongoing First World War, a point which Adam Parkes makes clear in his discussion of the prosecution:

> the ignoble ends to which Lawrence had put his mastery in the use of words were quite at odds with the righteous cause of war; in subverting the war effort, Lawrence was helping to send British soldiers to their graves. These arguments must have influenced Judge Dickinson, whose son had been killed in France shortly before the trial.[1]

The novel, in Parkes's reading, presents a form of morality incommensurate with the official British, Christian morality being mobilized against the perceived immorality and barbarism of the German aggressors: *The Rainbow* is then caught up in an anti-German legal agenda, testifying to the absence of a concerted effort to police literature itself but rather those articles which promoted values counter to the war effort and British identity.

DOI: 10.4324/9781003202509-1

But, on a closer inspection, the forms of legislation that maintained this identity are themselves implicated in the same cultural investments as those that seek to police literary obscenity. In the case of the offence of impersonating an officer of the British army, the law tasks itself with distinguishing and maintaining the veracity of a subject's symbolic mandate, the degree to which the subject's claims to a certain position within the Symbolic have been verified and thereby the law is safeguarding the institutional power that grants the subject the authority to exercise the privileges concomitant with that position: in short, it is a truth claim put into jeopardy by the simulacrum. The law's duty in this case is to maintain the appearance of the natural rights and privileges that the institution of the army claims for those subjects under its name and authority. In the case of the Trading with the Enemy Act 1914, we are dealing with a different kind of verification, namely who is an ally and who is the enemy. In the case of corporations, a legal fiction would usually be operative, whereby the corporation, and not the subjects who operate under the name of that corporation, functions as a legal subject. The Act allowed for the legal practice called lifting the corporate veil, wherein this fiction was erased, and the subjects operating under the name of the corporation were now scrutinized for enemy affiliations and liable for censure if found guilty.[2] In the case of this Act, we have the willing suspension of a legal fiction, a lifting of the veil, in the name of discerning the enemy operating surreptitiously underneath: one fiction, the corporation as a legal subject, is replaced by another, the enemy operating underneath and through fiction. In this understanding of the law, fictions, both literary and legal, are the privilege of peacetime; wartime law gave itself the duty of policing the signifier in order to distinguish between the British truth and the enemy: the foreign simulacrum. So, while Parkes is right to discern a wider context to the prosecution of Lawrence's text, the investments operative within that context remain. The simulacrum, of which the literary text is one example, poses a threat to the truth, to true and natural British values. Where the literary text distinguishes itself from these other forms of simulacrum is the degree to which the sexual element of the simulacrum becomes apparent.

The hearing was short: Methuen's representative pleaded guilty to the charges claiming ignorance of the obscene content of the novel. According to *The Telegraph*'s description of events, the publisher 'extremely regretted that they should have published the book' and that '[t]hey had never seen Mr Lawrence, but dealt with him though an agent'.[3] The agent had assured the publisher that any offending passages had been rewritten or expurgated, and the text had been published on good faith that this was the case.[4] This ignorance could not act as a defence to the charge, and the publisher was fined £10 10s, and the 1,011 copies of *The Rainbow* that had been seized were destroyed.

The prosecution and judge made a decision, in 'the public interest', to make statements on the nature of the text's obscenity, despite Methuen's admission of guilt rendering these statements superfluous. This excessive gesture, an incitement to discourse called forth by the literary text, indicates more at work here than a misunderstanding on the part of Methuen. Herbert Musker, speaking for the prosecution, declared that:

> To him personally it was a matter for the most profound regret that it should have been necessary for the protection of public morals and public decency in literary productions to bring this disgusting, detestable and pernicious work under the notice of the Court. Although there might not be an obscene word to be found in the book, it was in fact a mass of obscenity of thought, idea, and action, wrapped up in language which in some quarters might be considered artistic and intellectual. It was difficult to understand how Messrs Methuen could have lent their great name to the publication of this bawdy volume.[5]

To state that a text is obscene in the absence of any obscene words indicates a particular relation to language. For the prosecution, language is figured as a wrapping or veil that obscures the 'mass' of the object, the truth of the text. This obscene mass is figured as a unity of thought, idea and action. By extension, these categories also function separately from language and can be understood independently from language. To use the term mass also alludes to a perceived materiality to this truth, further asserting it as extra-discursive. A zone beyond language is being posited, and this zone is also figured as the place of truth. Musker also introduces a distinction between readers: there are some who would confuse the text's language as 'artistic and intellectual'. Those that concentrate on the language of the text, the argument would seem to follow, would miss the truth below or beyond: these subjects are by proxy stained with the same obscenity and coded as potential enemies to Britain. The law is presented as that which can see or read through language, witness the truth and return to language in order to name that truth. However, the limits of this hermeneutics are also apparent: in order to perform this reading, in order to produce the truth of the text, the specific material of the text must be ignored. To reject the specific words of the text is to offer no evidence for the claims being made. This practice is then based on a constitutive disavowal of the nature of the object it wishes to assess. Added to this problem is also the inability of the prosecution to name the truth it has witnessed after its unveiling. This mass is 'disgusting, detestable and pernicious' but lacks any description beyond its effects. At the same time, it is claiming access to a truth beyond language, the discourse of the prosecution reinstates the limits of language in being unable to say what it has seen. Here, the law is figured as a discourse of truth but one which must deny its own existence as discourse. This exceptional position produces an extra-discursive realm that the law can perceive and report. But the law confronts its limit at the point it is asked to bear witness, to speak the truth. Truth here functions both as the goal of speech but also as its absolute limit, an impossibility that is linked to a form of sexuality that produces disgust.

One aspect of Musker's statement that can further elucidate the way in which the law produces its claims to truth is the emphasis upon the proper name. It is the 'great name' of Methuen that is here condemned for having not properly policed itself. The name of Methuen should have functioned as a bulwark against obscenity but has failed in its duty to the public. Therefore, the name of Methuen, what that names beyond itself, has been brought into doubt. What the trial witnesses then is a crisis of the proper name, a crisis that requires the law to intervene and suture this rupture that has emerged between the symbolic/historical meaning of the name and the meaning of the actions taken by those working under the name. In this way, the law can be said to be profoundly invested and policing the signifier whilst also disavowing its own dependency upon it: when interrogating the literary text, the law disavows its interest in language, claiming access to an obvious truth exterior to it, but in regards to maintaining the meaning of the name 'Methuen', it is also attesting to a keen interest in the workings of language. This interest in the proper name is also apparent in the judge, Sir John Dickinson's, subsequent statement: he had

> never read anything more disgusting than this book, and how it could ever have passed through Messrs Methuen's hands he failed to understand. It was greatly to be regretted that a firm of old standing and the highest repute, whose name on the title-page of a book justified anyone taking it into their home, should allow their reputation to be soiled, as it undoubtedly had been. It was appalling to think of the harm that such a book might have done. It was utter filth; nothing else would describe it.[6]

Methuen's name is here figured as a guarantee against obscenity. The role of the publisher, according to Dickinson, is the policing of the domestic sphere, the proper name is put in service of property relations, and by extension, the obscene text is perceived as a threat to those relations. What is at stake in this trial is not only the obscenity of the text itself but also the ways and means by which the space in which the text is disseminated is taxonomized and policed. Key to this maintenance is the proper place of sexuality: the presence of sex where it is not meant to be, where it cannot be surveyed, measured and managed is the cause of much of the anxiety in these statements. Methuen's duty is then to help in this production of sexually stratified spaces and police the potentially disruptive forms of sexuality a text can contain. The 'high repute' of the name comes from its history of having been concomitant with this disciplinary function.

In Dickinson's statement, the title of the book is subordinated to the name of the publisher, the proper name of the publisher thus places both the title and the author of the book within a certain interpretive horizon that signifies the limits of the text's meaning and thus the safety of the reader and the domestic setting in which the reading takes place: but, *The Rainbow* has been perceived to transgress this limit and introduce an excess of filth and sexuality into a zone previously perceived as clean. What is at stake in this case is the failure of the publisher to correspond to the perceived meaning of its own name, an imbalance between the actions of the legal subject of Methuen and the reputation bestowed upon it by the law. As a result, the proper name is 'soiled' with the filth that is perceived in the text itself. *The Rainbow* thus enacts a reversal of the disciplinary function of the proper name. If the name of Methuen on a text signifies that all that comes under this name is sanitary and stabilizing; in this case, the 'utter filth' of the text has come to infect the name of Methuen, harming their reputation. The law's function here is then an act of public hygiene, the protection of public health and the suturing of the name of Methuen to its proper place within public discourse and thus restoring the performative magic of both the law and the institution of publishing.

Methuen's name functions not only as a guarantee against obscenity but also names a duty to the very function of guaranteeing. The name Methuen names a duty to those that live under the name, those legal subjects who work for the publishing house and the readers of the texts produced under that name. A certain responsibility is demanded for the maintenance of the name's meaning. Jacques Derrida in *Sauf Le Nom* identifies this duty as stemming from

> ... what the name supposes to name beyond itself, the nameable beyond the name, the unnameable nameable. As if it was necessary both to save the name, and to save everything except the name, *save the name* [sauf le nom], as if it was necessary to lose the name in order to save what bears the name, or that towards which one goes through the name. But to lose the name is not to attack it, to destroy it or wound it. On the contrary to lose the name is quite simply to respect it: as name.[7]

The nameable beyond the name denotes a truth beyond the limits of language, perceivable but unnameable. But a tension emerges here: is the name a product of the unnameable truth or is the pull of this truth dependent upon the instance of the name? This question repeats the anxiety located above in regard to the law's disavowed investment in the nature of language. The name of Methuen must be saved from obscenity, but this investment in the sanctity of the name betrays the malleability of the name itself. The stability of the truth beyond its name is brought into doubt not only by Methuen's actions but also by the possibility of intervention on the part of the law. In the very act of saving the name, the truth which that name is supposed to maintain is troubled, the proper name loses its privileged position and is reduced to the status of another signified in a differential and arbitrary position in relation to all other signifiers.[8] Any attempt to save the name also endangers the truth that the name protects, soiling its perceived purity. But Derrida also notes that the loss of the name can also strengthen the duty to that which the name was supposed to protect. What emerges in the process of saving the name is a clearer and codified definition of the duties incumbent upon the proper name of Methuen. The decision of the publisher to accept responsibility without defence performs a suturing of the gap that has emerged between the name and the subjects it names: the fantasy of realm beyond the name is maintained by the enunciation of the duty to protect it. The name is thus returned to its proper place, and the truth it names beyond itself can be assumed and enjoyed. But what is absent in Derrida's analysis is that even though the name is saved, during this process of suturing, another act of naming takes place. What is named are the conditions of possibility for the name to perform its specific political/disciplinary function. In other words, power not only speaks in this process but is also named. It is at this point that the function of the truth that the name names beyond itself is also named. By the very fact of intervention and the labour required to maintain the proper meaning of the proper name, the universality and neutrality of the name is lost, and the ideological function of its meaning can be perceived. The conditions of possibility of an extra-discursive zone of truth beyond the signifier are thus routed in specific power relations and techniques of control which are made apparent during the trial and the methods of maintenance operative within it. I will argue that these forms of maintenance have a specific political function: namely, the regulation and production of heteronormative subjectivities and the forms of enjoyment incumbent upon them.[9]

The maintenance of the proper name facilitates the reading practices of the trial: the truth of the text, what it names, is only apparent once the proper name of Methuen is in place. We can also see this dependency on names and titles in the trial's investment in Chapter 13 of *The Rainbow*, entitled 'Shame'. And it is upon this title that the prosecution and the judge base their reading of the text. After declaring themselves as unaware of the text's obscenity, Methuen is accused of having not properly read the text. Musker commented in his statement that 'it was a remarkable fact that two members of the firm read a certain chapter to which particular exception was taken without conceiving the suggestion it contained'.[10] Here again, the prosecution's discourse is telling of a particular relationship to language dependent both on the proper name and the unnameable. The literary text, according to the prosecution's argument, functions as a container of specific and stable truths which a proper reader can extract and consider in isolation. The truth extracted from the container can be considered as separate from the container itself and therefore can be judged as obscene even if the container, the very language of the text, gives no indication of this obscenity. But the very reticence to name the chapter, instead referring to it as 'a certain chapter' belies the neutral relation to language that this reading depends upon. The same reticence is apparent in the absence of specificity in the apparently obvious 'suggestion'. The suggestion is obvious, and the absence of its perception demands to be remarked upon, but what exactly it suggests cannot be named. This refusal to name the obscene would seem to indicate a form of repression operative in this discourse, as if the relation to language that allows Musker to perform the role of assigning the proper name also forbids him from naming it as such: the proper name of the obscene content of Lawrence's text is deferred.

A similar dynamic is at play in Judge Dickinson's condemnation of Methuen and the 'Shame' chapter. Dickinson, bemused by Methuen's claims to not have read anything obscene in the chapter, claimed that Methuen 'could not have read very intelligently, looking at the name of the chapter- "Shame"'.[11] Here again, the practice of reading properly amounts to the reading of the proper name, this time, the title of the chapter. The title 'Shame' is read as naming the content of the chapter and labels it obscene. We have then a reading practice that is dependent upon a chain of proper names, beginning with the name of the publisher and continuing on to the name of the chapter. Only with these names in their proper place and having a fixed and agreed upon meaning can the content of the text appear to the reader. But once again, the word 'shame' is a deferral away from the name of the sexual content that the law has found obscene. Parkes argues that the term shame functions in the trial as a cypher for homosexuality and specifically to the bathing scene between Ursula and Winifred in the chapter.[12] In my argument, this would continue to be the case, but I wish to add to Parkes's account by delineating the specific relation to language that is being used by the law in order to categorize and regulate sexuality. A double bind emerges here in relation to the proper name: it is required to remain in place in order for the obscene to be recognized. However, that obscenity can also not be directly named: it is obvious but only relayed in coded form. If, following Derrida, the law has a duty to the unnameable beyond the name, then we can also see operative here the unnameable quality of the obscene, connected to queer sexuality. We have both a good unnameable, the truth and an obscene form of the unnameable that appears to function as the truth's opposite and is connected to sexuality.

There is, then, operative in the court's reading practice, an investment in the proper name: that investment, as Derrida points out, relates to a fantasized zone of truth beyond the name that remains certain but also unnameable. It is towards the maintenance of this fantasy that the prosecution of the text takes place. Another unnameable quantity is also operating in the trial, connected to the meaning of Lawrence's text, obscenity and homosexuality. To understand this other, obscene aspect, of the proper name, I will now have recourse to Lacan's discussion of the proper name in *Seminar XII*:

> it is in the fact that it is irreplaceable, namely that it can be lacking, that it suggests at the level of lack, the level of the hole, and that it is it not qua individual that I am called Jacques Lacan, but qua something which may be lacking, which means that this name will be for what? To cover over another lack. The proper name, as one might say, is a movable function [...] designed to fill the holes, to be a shutter, to close it down, to give it a false appearance of suture.[13]

That the proper name is needed indicates that it can be lost. The subject who invests in the proper name, who assigns it the value of being 'irreplaceable', does so according to a perceived lack. The object that is assigned a name, in this case, the subject called Lacan, is not given that name according to some characteristic inherent in the object, but in order to appease a structural requirement of language, the requirement to exist within the symbolic as a name, a placeholder. It is this compulsion that suggests the covering of 'another lack', a lack at the level of the signifier itself. The proper name is thus a 'moveable function' giving a 'false appearance' of suture. The trial, in its acknowledgment of the split between the name of Methuen and the actions of the firm, attests to a failure in this moveable function and the disintegration, however temporary, of the suture itself. This failure of the suture, as is apparent in the trial, is presented in terms of anxieties regarding sexuality and contagion of the domestic sphere, as if sexuality, and particularly in feminine and queer forms, threatened the collapse of the domestic itself.

This lack that the proper name masks is not, I would like to argue, a prediscursive realm of primal sexual instinct as it might appear in Lacan's above description, but rather is an effect of the enunciation of the proper name itself. If the name announces a truth beyond itself, then it also, at this very moment, effects its own impossibility, the denial of this truth ever being actualized. In other words, the Symbolic of the law, its discourse, is dependent upon an Imaginary, fantasized, beyond in order to bestow consistency upon itself. But what is also apparent within the discourse of the trial, is an unnameable kernel of obscenity operative in this discourse, one that is repeatedly elided but always returns. This traumatic Real of the Law also functions as the support for the forms of reading required to maintain its functioning which in turn preserves the consistency of the proper name.

Another way to distinguish between these two forms of the unnameable is to distinguish between the two forms of singularity that each implies. In the terms of the Symbolic, the proper name indicates a given signifier's place in a differential relation with other signifiers. Entrance into the Symbolic for the subject bestows that subject with identity only in relation to other subjects with the big Other operating as the guarantor for these relations. Thus, the subject, through language, is able to mean and understand. It is from these relations that legal subjects can be discerned, and rights can be conceived and produced for them. This difference is limited however as they are different only in so far as they are the same, and under the same name and the same shared fantasy of the big Other's consistency. But another form of singularity emerges at the same time, a form of singularity that resists reduction to the level of the signified. If entrance into the symbolic is to enter into an economy of signification in order to bestow identity, this other form is wholly incommensurate with this economy. As Joan Copjec describes it, 'in language and yet more than language, the subject is a cause for which no signifier can account. Not because she transcends the signifier but because she inhabits it as limit'.[14] The subject exceeds the capacity of the signifier to name its entire being, some part of its existence is always missed in its enunciation, remains unnameable.

Lee Edelman identifies this form of singularity, that which remains unspeakable, with queer sexuality. As indeed do the judges and prosecution when they confront Ursula's desire for Winifred in *The Rainbow*. For Edelman, because this unspeakable form of singularity is heterogeneous to the Symbolic economy, it is perceived as a threat and an embodiment of death. The queer comes to embody both those aspects that Freud identifies as causing the forgetting of the proper name: death and sexuality.[15] As Edelman argues:

> As the constancy of a pressure both alien and internal to the logic of the Symbolic, as the inarticulable surplus that dismantles the subject from within, the death drive names what the queer, in the order of the social, is called forth to figure: the negativity opposed to every form of social viability.[16]

Here, the double meaning of queer, both a deviation from a general norm and a collective name for forms of non-normative sexuality, is mobilized by Edelman by having the queer stand both as the surplus of the system itself, and the subject whose sexual practices and, by extension, his own being, comes to be coded as the bearer of that surplus. The queer here functions as an embodiment of the death drive, as a threat to 'every form of social viability', that is the very grounds upon which intersubjective connections. The guarantor of these relations, the safeguard of the Symbolic and the forms of fantasy required to maintain the impression that the Symbolic is a unified field, is the law itself. Using Edelman's analysis, one can begin to understand the investment the law has in policing and destroying dissident sexuality, whether in the form of punishing sexual dissidents or censoring representations of deviant sexual behaviour: those subjects and practices function as the means by which the presence of this surplus of non-meaning operative in the symbolic itself is projected onto the obscene text or queer subject and subsequently scapegoated, a ritual cleansing of the presence of death within the proper name.

But here emerges a fundamental problem in Edelman's analysis: in apprehending the Symbolic as a monolithic and ahistorical phenomenon that always finds its enemy in the figure of the queer, Edelman thus essentializes both the Symbolic and the queer. This essentialism is problematic for a number of reasons. First, it presumes that non-heteronormative practices have always been coded as detrimental to the functioning of the polis and always will: both of these contentions have been challenged by Foucault in all three volumes of *The History of Sexuality*, wherein he describes the vast difference between homosexual practices in modern Europe as compared to Ancient Greek and Rome. More recently, Jasbir Puar has convincingly demonstrated the ability for contemporary Western colonialism to co-opt queer subjects into its project. Homo-nationalism for Puar names the process by which White American queerness can function a form of 'sexual-exceptionalism' that differentiates these patriotic queers from non-White queer subjects who are those coded as potential threats to the nation.[17] In Puar's analysis, the queer itself can be allocated a proper name, a duty to conform to a particular position within the Symbolic. This process, along with the increasingly tolerant position, taken towards queer subjects within liberal nations since the publication of Edelman's text would seem to trouble his assertion that the queer subject and his *jouissance* are essentially on the side of death.[18]

Which brings us to another problem in coding the queer as an embodiment of death: the problem of sexual difference. Edelman makes no distinction between female and male enjoyment, only heteronormative and queer. In doing so, he manages to elide the difficult concept of feminine *jouissance* which we find in Lacan's later work. This distinction between phallic and feminine *jouissance* will be discussed later in this chapter, but for now, it is sufficient to assert that in Lacan and his later followers, the feminine form of enjoyment has, like the queer in Edelman, been posited as a defacto transgressive form of enjoyment that escapes codification by the Symbolic. If we are to take this link between queerness and death seriously in an analysis of the trial, as the discourse of trial itself demands, the reading must remain attentive to the vicissitudes of queerness that continue to shift depending on a multitude of discourses that intersect in order to produce a queer subject and code that subject's enjoyment as useful or transgressive, on the side of life or on the side of death.

Despite these reservations, queerness, queer enjoyment and death are being linked in this trial. It is also clear that depictions of queer sexual practices are perceived as a threat to the population of England at this time. The specificity of this threat cannot be enunciated in the discourse of the trial, however. This is an impossibility inherent within legal discourse itself. The law's structural investment in a fantasy of a realm of truth beyond the signifier necessarily forces it to confront its own inconsistency, its own existence as language, its affinity to the simulacrum it wishes to police. As I have argued above, the discourse of the law is reliant upon the proper name to perform the work of identifying and ultimately supressing obscenity. But, in doing so, the proper name is troubled in such a way as to stain it with a potential obscenity, creating a momentary crisis, wherein what the name signifies is undecidable.

This link between the queer, shame and the literary text has further and more historically specific implications linking back to my discussion on the crisis of investiture operative within the law, a crisis only worsened by the onset of war. Eric Stanley argues that the emergence of the queer as a destabilizing force, the queer as enemy, is a product of the emergence of liberal democracy. He argues that:

> the human, the "something" [...] within the context of the liberal democracy, names rights-bearing subjects, or those who can stand as subjects before the law. The human, then, makes the nothing not only possible but necessary. Following this logic, the work of death, of the death that is already nothing, not quite human, binds the categorical (mis)recognition of humanity. The human, then, resides in the space of life and under the domain of rights, whereas the queer inhabits the place of compromised personhood and the zone of death. As perpetual and axiomatic threat

> to the human, the queer is the negated double of the subject of liberal democracy.[19]

In the absence of the sovereign, under whose name a subject could become recognized by the law as a legal subject, the queer is produced to function as the figure against whom the law is set. The heteronormative subject gains consistency and legal rights by virtue of renouncing any potential identification with the queer subject and, instead, identifying with his status as a legal subject. But this identification with the law and the privileges and powers it allows is predicated upon a fundamental misrecognition, facilitated by fantasy, of the law and the human as stable and natural categories that do not depend upon the queer as its obscene double for the appearance of their constancy. Other psychoanalytic thinkers highlight the degree to which sexuality puts into question the distinction between heteronormativity and queer as distinct categories: the proscriptions placed upon sex, the necessary practices to prove one's heteronormativity, testify to a pre-existing form of sexuality that requires the intervention of the law to force it into a normative form. This is a point that Alenka Zupancic makes in *What Is Sex?* She argues that the normative transition from polymorphous perversity towards genital sexual organization constitutes a perversion of the sexual in and of itself:

> This unification is always a somehow forced and artificial [and] it is never really fully achieved or accomplished, which is to say that it never transforms the sexual drive into an organic unity, with all its components ultimately serving one and the same purpose. "Normal," "healthy" human sexuality is thus a paradoxical, artificial naturalization of the originally denatured drives [...]. One could even say that human sexuality is "sexual" (and not simply "reproductive") precisely insofar as the unification at stake, the tying of all the drives to one single purpose, never really works, but allows for different partial drives to continue their circular, self-perpetuating activity.[20]

Genitally organized heterosexuality, the apparently normal aim of sexual development in the subject, is itself an artifice, a fiction constructed from the partial drives operative within the child. Being constructed from this multitude of closed circuits, the intended fixing of the subject's sexuality towards a normative object necessarily fails. It is precisely in the domain of fantasy that this failure is elided. The fantasy of the sexual relation thus facilitates the belief in a normal object of desire as well as allowing the partial drives to continue their perpetuation unheeded. What is required for its maintenance, and particularly in the absence of the sovereign threat of violence, is a performative dimension in which practices coded as heterosexual are performed in order to testify to one's heteronormativity. Failure to perform these practices thus codes a subject's enjoyment as transgressive and testifies to the sexual non-relation. The non-relation then requires the intervention of the law and the violence of the law in order to suture the rip in the cultural Imaginary caused by this transgression. In Zupancic's model, as opposed to Edelman's, we retain the same transgressive dimension of the queer but avoid the accusation of essentialism: the drive is constitutive of sex in all its dimensions.

The *jouissance* of the drive can thus be made to work for the structure it erodes. Derrida in *Archive Fever* is particularly attuned to this dynamic. He argues that:

> radical destruction can again be reinvested in another logic, in the inexhaustible economistic resource of an archive which capitalizes everything, even that which ruins it or radically contests its power: radical evil can be of service, infinite destruction can be reinvested in a theodicy, the devil can also serve to justify.[21]

The perpetual work of the drive is put to work in the name of the law in the form of an archival process which sets itself a duty to collate all available data upon the forces that threaten the fantasmatic basis of order: perpetual surveillance of potentially dissident enjoyment. The psychoanalytic and the biopolitical converge in this instance of an overlap with this archival death drive and the panoptical schemes of surveillance described by Foucault, wherein sexuality emerges as an object of knowledge and study. Jodi Dean argues that it is in fact this very drive that fuels the apparatuses of biopower.[22] Key amongst these subjects, according to Foucault, were homosexuals and women, those whose mutual enjoyment was coded as both an object of knowledge and a threat. These two forms of enjoyment, merging in the unspoken figure of the lesbian, are archived by the law in this trial under the name of shame. The lesbian takes on the dimension of ~~The~~ Woman's obscene double, an impossible object of desire but one whom cannot be accessed, who has no desire to seduce and can thus promise no form of knowledge beyond the signifier.

It is, then, worth returning to the function of the term shame within the trial. The shame that names Lawrence's chapter, that functions for the judge and prosecution as an oblique, name for queer sexuality, requires not only censure but also a deferral of the affect it names: it is as if the (im)proper name has put into question the propriety of the proper name itself. To understand this link between shame, the proper name and queer sexuality, it is beneficial to interrogate that particular affect in a psychoanalytic context. In *Imagine There's No Woman*, Copjec argues that shame attests to a fundamental rupture in the fantasmatic fabric of the subject:

> Shame is awakened not when one looks at oneself, or those whom one cherishes, through another's eyes, but when one suddenly perceives a lack in the Other. At this moment the subject no longer experiences herself as the fulfilment of the Other's desire, as the center of the world, which now shifts away from her slightly, causing a distance to open within the subject

> herself. This distance is not that "superegoic" one which produces a feeling of guilt and burdens one with an uncancelable debt to the Other, but is, on the contrary, that which wipes out the debt. In shame, unlike guilt, one experiences one's visibility, but there is no external Other who sees, since shame is proof that the Other does not exist.[23]

Shame signifies the failure of the subject to perform the requisite practices that testify to their normality, their proper place, thus bringing into question the naturalness of those practices. In their failure, the performative dimension of power appears artificial, as a fictional relation to the world. The law's intervention then signifies not the absolute presence of the big Other but rather its impotence. Shame is the result of the failure of seduction to elicit the truth beyond the signifier desired by the subject: proof that ~~The~~ Woman does not exist. Ursula's brief sexual encounter with Winifred elicits shame in its reader, in the psychoanalytic sense that it elicits an encounter with the non-existence of ~~The~~ Woman. This shame demands legal intervention.

Examining again the mobilization of the term shame in the trial, one can see how it operates through deferral onto another subject or object until it is transformed into guilt. Guilt can be transfigured into a numerical value and an accepted debt repaid. The act of reparation attests to not only the lifting of the debt but also to the existence and legitimacy of the creditor, the law itself: it is an act that reinstates the Other into the dimension of the subject's desire, proof that the Other exists and the law, in turn, is legitimate. Dickinson reads the unnameable presence of death within the pages of the chapter entitled Shame. This, in turn, institutes a crisis in representation, whereby the obscenity alluded to cannot enter the discourse of the law, testifying to the law's impotence and discursive limits. The cause for this crisis of the proper name is placed upon the publishers and their failure to uphold the disciplinary function of their name. The subjects operating under that name accept responsibility for the failure of the proper name and in doing so allow the law to locate this failure in transgressive legal subject's decisions, Metheun and Lawrence, as opposed to language itself. Thus, shame, which testifies to the absence of the sexual relation, is transfigured into guilt, which produces a debt to the Other, thus reasserting the existence of the Other and the sexual relation.

Notably, the subject who pays the debt is not the author as the law is more concerned with the subject of the enunciation rather than the enunciating subject. Robert Spoo, commenting on the transition from previous obscenity statutes towards the 1854 act and the subsequent Hicklin ruling, comments that:

> libel actions, typically begun in personam, often concluded with a judgement or settlement in rem, requiring the destruction of the offending res, the stock of books containing the injurious falsehood. In rem solutions disabled the communications circuit by simply removing the signal.[24]

By disabling the communications circuit, the concomitant circulation of the death drive and its concomitant *jouissance* could also be curtailed. With the law restored and the proper name saved from the shame of its own impotence, the only outstanding testament to this crisis was the text. Dickinson's order for the remaining copies of *The Rainbow* to be destroyed constitutes the erasure of the form of enjoyment the text was perceived to embody. But this process of destruction, and the archiving of this project in the legal records, attests to the presence of the destructive drive operative within the law itself.

The surviving archival residue of the trial is slight. Beyond the ledger detailing the litigant and penalty and the small amount of media coverage given to the trial, there is little to testify to the failure of the proper name that took place within it. The trial is also the only one in this book wherein the discourse of literary criticism will not be mobilized in the name of the obscene text in order to attest to its value. The absence of this discourse allows the law to act as the sole discourse of truth and code the text as an embodiment of the death drive it must necessarily fail to acknowledge in itself. The increasing presence of the discourse of literary criticism and an attendant increase in media coverage will complicate this process of naming considerably. But even without resistance from either literary criticism, or the subjects' accused, the process by which the law reads the literary text, decides upon its truth and ultimately destroys it, leaves traces of a fundamental ambivalence brought about by the literary text.

Notes

1 Adam Parkes, *Modernism and the Theater of Censorship*, (Oxford: Oxford University Press, 1996), p. 5.

2 The key case under this act was *Daimler Co Ltd v Continental Tyre and Rubber Co (Great Britain) Ltd*, wherein the House of Lords decided that the fact that the majority of shareholders in Continental Tyre and Rubber Co Ltd's were German residents constituted the company as the enemy and all subjects who traded with them would be liable for prosecution under the act.

3 'An Objectionable Novel: Messrs Metheun Summoned', in *The Daily Telegraph*, 15 November 1915, p. 15.

4 Lawrence did attempt to comply with demands to remove phrases from the novel that could be interpreted as obscene. He refused to substantively omit larger passages and paragraphs however. In a letter on the subject, Lawrence wrote that:

> [t]he passages and paragraphs marked I cannot alter. There is nothing offensive in them, beyond the very substance they contain, and that is no more offensive than that of all the rest of the novel. The libraries won't object to the book any less, or approve of it any more, if these passages are cut out.

David H. Lawrence, *The Letters of D.H. Lawrence*, Volume 2, ed. George Zytaruk and James T. Boulton, (Cambridge: Cambridge University Press, 1981), pp. 369–370. There is a striking similarity between Lawrence's faith in the substance of the text not being effected by the language of the text itself and the prosecution's belief in the truth of the text being found beyond or underneath the language of the text.

5 *Telegraph*, p. 17.

6 Ibid.

7 Jacques Derrida, 'Sauf Le Nom', trans. John P. Leavey, Jr., in *On The Name*, ed. Thomas Dutoit, (Stanford, CA: Stanford University Press, 1995), pp. 35–89, p. 58.

8 Derrida is aware of this double movement and its attendant anxieties: 'If the name never belongs originarily and rigorously to s/he who receives it, it also no longer belongs from the very first moment to s/he who gives it' (Ibid. p. 59).

9 In the section of *The Psychopathology of Everyday Life* entitled 'Forgetting of Proper Names', Freud recalls his own forgetting of the name Signorelli. The forgotten name, Freud argues, undergoes 'a division into two pieces' (Sigmund Freud, 'The Psychopathology of Everyday Life', in The *Standard Edition of The Complete Psychological Works of Sigmund, Freud: Volume VI*, ed. and Trans. James Strachey, (London: Hogarth Press, 1981), p. 6.). The proper name is re-found through the discovery of other syllables in Freud's previous conversation with his friend and the associations that his discourse aroused in him. What is important to note is this splitting of the name has as its root cause in the desire to repress something other than the name. Freud names that which was repressed as 'the theme of death and sexuality' (p. 6) that would have emerged in Freud's conversation had the repression not taken place.

If the actions of Methuen in publishing *The Rainbow* constitute a forgetting of the name, it would imply that a form of repression has taken place, namely the same theme of death and sexuality that Freud locates as the cause is also apparent in Lawrence's text, a text that takes great interest in both death and sexuality and the ways in which they interact. The forgetting of the proper name can then be designated as an effect of the text itself on the discourse of the trial. If the law is the protector and guarantor of the proper name, then death and sexuality constitute a threat to its proper functioning.

There is another aspect to the trial that is not apparent in Freud's account of the proper name. The return of the name to its proper place also requires an act of repression. In this case, the text itself must be condemned and taken out of circulation and disowned by the publisher. The process of suture that the trial enacts requires that death and sexuality also be repressed, to return them to the unnameable. But as the trial also demonstrates, the unnameable beyond the name is also what the law depends upon to produce a duty to the proper name.

10 *Telegraph*, p. 17.

11 Ibid.

12 Parkes, *Modernism*, p. 28. Parkes also argues that the connection between the word shame was predominantly used as a cypher for male homosexuality and that this trial's use of the term in relation to lesbianism is relatively anomalous.

13 Jacques Lacan, *Seminar XII: Crucial Problems for Psychoanalysis*, trans. Cormac Gallagher, p. 50.

14 Joan Copjec, *Read My Desire*, (London: MIT Press, 1994), p. 209.

15 Freud, *Psychopathology*, p. 5.

16 Lee Edelman, *No Future: Queer Theory and the Death Drive*, (London: Duke University Press, 2004), p. 9.

17 Jasbir Puar, *Terrorist Assemblages: Homonationalism in Queer Times*, (London: Duke University Press, 2007), p. 34.

18 Edelman's queer is definitively male, troubling any attempt to figure queer enjoyment as fully heterogenous from the phallic *jouissance* of the heteronormative subject.

19 Eric Stanley, 'Near Life, Queer Death Overkill and Ontological Capture', in *Social Text*, Vol. 29, No. 2 (107), Summer 2011, pp. 1–19, p. 7.

20 Alenka Zupančič, *What Is Sex?* (London: MIT Press, 2017), p. 9.

21 Jacques Derrida, *Archive Fever: A Freudian Impression*, trans. Eric Prenowitz, (London: The University of Chicago Press, 1995), p. 18.

22 Jodi Dean, 'Drive as the Structure of Biopolitics', in *Krisis*, Vol. 2, 2010, pp. 1–15, p. 10.

23 Joan Copjec, *Imagine There's No Woman: Women and Sublimation*, (London: MIT Press, 2002), p. 128.

24 Robert Spoo, *Modernism and the Law*, (London: Bloomsbury, 2018), p. 13.

Bibliography

'An Objectionable Novel: Messrs Metheun Summoned', in *The Daily Telegraph*, November 15 1915.

Copjec, Joan, *Imagine There's No Woman: Women and Sublimation*, (London: MIT Press, 2002).

———, *Read My Desire*, (London: MIT Press, 1994).

Dean, Jodi, 'Drive as the Structure of Biopolitics', in *Krisis*, Vol. 2, 2010, pp. 1–15.

Derrida, Jacques, *Archive Fever: A Freudian Impression*, trans. Eric Prenowitz, (London: The University of Chicago Press, 1995).

———, 'Sauf Le Nom', trans. John P. Leavey, Jr., in *On the Name*, ed. Thomas Dutoit, (Stanford, CA: Stanford University Press, 1995), pp. 35–88.

Edelman, Lee, *No Future: Queer Theory and the Death Drive*, (London: Duke University Press, 2004).

Freud, Sigmund, 'The Psychopathology of Everyday Life', in The *Standard Edition of the Complete Psychological Works of Sigmund, Freud: Volume VI*, ed. and trans. James Strachey, (London: Hogarth Press, 1981), pp. 1–289.

Kittler, Friedrich, *Discourse Networks1800/1900*, trans. Chris Cullens and Michael Metteer, (Stanford, CA: Stanford University Press, 1992).

Kochis, Matthew J. and Heather L. Lusty (ed.), *Modernists at Odds: Reconsidering Joyce and Lawrence*, (Miami: University of Florida Press, 2015).

Lacan, Jacques, *Seminar XII: Crucial Problems for Psychoanalysis*, trans. Cormac Gallagher, http://www.lacaninireland.com/web/wp-content/uploads/2010/06/12-Crucial-problems-for-psychoanalysis.pdf.

Lawrence, David H., *The Letters of D.H. Lawrence*, Volume 2, ed. George Zytaruk and James T. Boulton, (Cambridge: Cambridge University Press, 1981), pp. 369–370.

Parkes, Adam, *Modernism and the Theater of Censorship*, (Oxford: Oxford University Press, 1996).

Puar, Jasbir, *Terrorist Assemblages: Homonationalism in Queer Times*, (London: Duke University Press, 2007).

Stanley, Eric, 'Near Life, Queer Death Overkill and Ontological Capture', in *Social Text* Vol. 29, No. 2 (107), Summer 2011, pp. 1–19.

Spoo, Robert, *Modernism and the Law*, (London: Bloomsbury, 2018).

Zupančič, Alenka, *What Is Sex?* (London: MIT Press, 2017).

2

THE LAW OF THE JUNGERL

When *Ulysses* was brought to trial during 1920–1921, the novel had yet to be finished. Chapters were appearing periodically in America through the *avant-garde* journal *The Little Review*, which was edited by two women: Jane Heap and Margaret Anderson. The journal had already garnered attention from censors before the trial of *Ulysses*. In October 1917, The United States Post Office seized copies of *The Little Review* containing Wyndham Lewis's short story 'Cantleman's Spring Mate'. Both sex and war, in Lewis's short story, are linked to an ecstatic death. And if it is the case that the text was censured solely on the grounds of America's imminent entry into the war, then its obscenity can be located not just in its representation of a lecherous soldier but on the linking of the war itself to sexuality and implicating both war and sexuality in the *jouissance* of the drive, thus bringing into question the national identities upon which the war was based. And, as we will come to see, the linkage between sex, gender and national identity will again emerge in the later *Little Review* trial in a different form.

Perhaps, more important than the censorship of Lewis's text is the subsequent reaction to it from leading modernists. Ezra Pound, a somewhat reluctant patron to *The Little Review*, was outraged to discover that the law that gave the Postal Service the remit to seize obscene literature, the Comstock laws, also included legislation aimed to curb the traffic of contraceptive devices.[1] In an essay published in *The Little Review* entitled 'The Classics Escape', Pound declared that he 'object[ed] to a law which doesn't keep the two issues distinct. AND a country which can't distinguish between the two is in a bloody rotten state of barbarism'.[2] Pound was particularly irked by Judge Hand's admittance that many texts that were considered at that time as 'classics' would probably be deemed obscene if published at that time. 'The classics', Hand argued, were 'immune' to the statute only by virtue of 'the sanction of age and fame and usually appeal to a comparatively limited number of readers'.[3] By arguing that supposed canonical works of

DOI: 10.4324/9781003202509-2

literature are only saved from the censor by convention rather than their intrinsic moral worth, Hand highlights the extent to which the law holds all literature potentially stained with obscenity. Pound interpreted Hand's lack of respect towards canonical literature to be a sign of the judge's illiteracy. These canonical texts, Pound argues, 'lifted mankind from savagery, and which from A.D. 1400 onward have gradually redeemed us from the darkness of medievalism'.[4] The classics, for Pound, serve as a disciplinary function, acting as a healthy supplement to mankind's inherently savage nature. The censorship of modern literature puts this process of cultivation in jeopardy as this supplement that maintains order and progress was being attacked by the legal apparatus of the nation.

We find a variation on Pound's arguments in Heap's account of the *Ulysses* trial. In her editorial piece in *The Little Review* entitled 'Art and the Law', Heap argues that there is a fundamental difference between the function of law and that of art:

> In a physical world laws have been made to preserve physical order. Laws cannot reach, nor have power over, any other realm. Art is and always has been the supreme Order. Because of this it is the only activity of man that has an eternal quality. Works of Art are the only permanent sign that man has existed. What legal genius to bring Law against Order![5]

For Pound and Heap, albeit in different ways, the work of art helps forge and maintain bonds between subjects: art is the means by which collective identity is produced. In a psychoanalytic sense, we could argue that, for Heap and Pound, art functions in much the same way as for Mathew Arnold, providing the co-ordinates for collective desire at the level of fantasy. This logic will form the basis of both the legal opposition to obscenity and the function of literary criticism in these trials.[6] The saving grace of the literary text is its utility, the uses it can be put to within a culture: literature's value here is its disciplinary potential. The work of art brings order and thus props up the fantasy of the sexual relation, of fixed meaning and identity. A fundamental antagonism emerges here between the law and the critic. Both discourses claim their object of study as a unifying force whilst accusing the other of attempting to curtail that order. We have in both positions the psychoanalytic phenomenon of transference, whereby the subject perceives a form of truth within the signifiers of their particular discourse. This investment in the law or literature as a discourse of truth signals a concomitant identity formed upon the truth content of the chosen discourse. These identities come under threat by the drive which constantly effaces the enjoyment in meaning that is identity: as in the previous trial, literature is once again an embodiment of the death drive, but here, we can see that the law too can be perceived as an embodiment of the same drive. Perhaps, both arguments, with slight amendments, help discern a particular instance of the drive at work within culture. What the law perceives is the radical threat of the Real that a literary text can produce. What Pound, Heap and Anderson perceive is the presence of the drive at the very core of the law itself, the masturbatory repetition that keeps within its own circuit disallowing any potential recoding that literature could offer. Both sides remain ignorant of the concomitancy of their insights due to the transference at play.

In regard to Lacan's graph that, due to the transference, each party is positing its discourse in the place of Φ, the father function, and as such, each argument reproduces the masculine structural formation of desire. As such, the figure of ~~The~~ Woman, *object petit a*, and the problem of feminine *jouissance* all pervade the unconscious of the trial of *The Little Review*. All three find their embodiment in the figure of the Young-Girl, upon whom both the prosecution and defence base their case. The Young-Girl will operate as the master signifier in whose name, the trial will be justified and the project of policing obscenity in general finds its legitimacy. As will be borne out in this chapter's analysis of the trial, the Young-Girl is itself a variation upon The Woman, which as we argued earlier is one of the Names-of-the-Father. These fantasmatic figures function as the grounds upon which law bases its claims to truth and provides cohesion within the ideological field of a given community. But, crucially, these fantasy figure bear no essential relation to the lived experiences of the subjects that they name; thus, their continued existence and the enjoyment they sustain are based upon the continual repression and elision of the lived experience of women.

The facts leading to the prosecution of *The Little Review* were as follows: in an attempt to find new subscribers for the financially ailing magazine, Heap sent unsolicited copies of the edition to many households in the state of New York. One of these copies was sent to the home of a New York lawyer.[7] The text fell into the hands of the lawyer's daughter who, after reading the journal alerted the offending article to her father, apparently offended and 'demanding that the magazine be prosecuted'. In response, the father sent the following letter to District Attorney of New York County, Edward Swan:

> Dear Sir,
>
> I enclose a copy under another cover—of a copy of 'The Little Review' which was sent to my daughter unsolicited. Please read the passages marked on pages 43, 45, 50 and 51. If such indecencies don't come within the provisions of the Postal Laws then isn't there some way in which the circulation of such things can be confined among the people who buy or subscribe to a publication of this kind? Surely there must be some way of keeping such 'literature' out of the homes of people who don't want it even if, in the interests of morality, there is no means of suppressing it.[8]

The letter reveals the anxieties surround the literary text but also the means of disseminating the text. The literary text and the increasingly efficient technology of the postal service are here tainted with the same suspicion of obscenity. Rachel Potter highlights the fact that the Postal Services of Europe and the

U.S. became the primary means for publishers of obscene texts to evade the laws surrounding the publishing of sexually explicit texts.[9] Friedrich Kittler in *Discourse Networks* also emphasizes that the increase in efficiency of postal services leads to concomitant loosening of national boundaries.[10] We have then a situation whereby the flows of information that the postal service facilitates become linked in the cultural imagination to the flow of obscene desires that threaten that culture and the identities formed national boundaries: in short, the presence of the other within the fantasied closed boundaries of the community. The father's desire to circumscribe the circulation of obscene literature occurs as a result of the domestic sphere, both his property and his nation, being breached by a foreign body intent on corrupting the bourgeois family and the masculine identity that it supports. Of course, he cannot phrase it this way because to do so would reveal the contingency of that identity upon the very *jouissance* that he perceives as its threat. Instead, the one at risk is his daughter, upon whom he projects his fantasy of Imaginary fullness. But the law cannot function on the singular young girl in question so a general fantasy figure that come to stand in for all young girls in the nation must be posited to justify prosecution. It is this figure of the Young-Girl, a fantasy formation projected onto the screen of women's bodies that the entire trial of *The Little Review* will come to revolve.

Swan, upon receiving the letter, assigned the complaint to Assistant District Attorney decided to ask the opinion of John Sumner, the head of the New York Society for the Suppression of Vice, the institution brought into existence by the Comstock laws for the policing of obscenity in the state.[11] The NYSSV was responsible for the majority of obscenity prosecutions in the state. In an article he penned for *The Dial*, Sumner described how the society went about prosecuting suspected peddlers of obscenity and attempted to justify the society's existence in relation to the prosecution of *The Little Review*. 'The New York Society for the Suppression of Vice', was, according to Sumner, 'an agency to receive the complaint of the ordinary citizen and be his proxy in enforcing the law'.[12] On most occasions, the NYSSV would have a member of the public purchase a prohibited text and then finance the prosecution of the text. The member of the public would not have to bear witness against the text. Instead, and this is probably due to the Hicklin test's emphasis on the vulnerable reader rather than the average reader, the defence, prosecution and judges would have to imagine the text's effect on the absent witness; in this case, the lawyer's daughter who read the *Nausicaa* chapter in *The Little Review*. Sumner defends this practice by appealing to the practicality of calling witnesses:

> Of course, John Doe could have been called in from the street and requested to act as complaining witness in *The Little Review* case, but John Doe would just as certainly have declined the honour because he had a family to support and his time was entirely taken up with the business which was his livelihood.[13]

Sumner's appeal to pragmatism discloses key anxieties and elides the facts of the case at hand. His ideal witness is male, but in this case, the offended witness was female. Sumner's fudging of the facts alludes to both the default phallic nature of the law as well as exposing the repressed and repressive dependency of male identity upon the feminine. The fact that the lawyer's daughter cannot testify is not only due to practicality but also performs the specific ideological function of removing any female lived experience from the trial; the definition of ~~The~~ Woman's response to the text will be decided by men. We can see in Sumner's statement the repressed element of the Young-Girl. It is she who supports 'John Doe', sustains his narcissistic identity and regulates his access to *jouissance*, not the other way around. The disciplinary institution of the family, 'his business' and 'his livelihood', by which we can insinuate his entire psychical reality, depend upon this anonymous and silent Young-Girl.

It is worth interrogating this figure of the Young-Girl as a discursive trope in order to distinguish it and its fantasmatic function from actual women and their lived experience. In their text *Preliminary Materials for a Theory of the Young Girl*, Tiqqun argues that after the First World War, the figure of the Young-Girl emerges as 'the model citizen as redefined by consumer society[...] in response to [...]revolutionary menace'.[14] The Young-Girl is invoked in order to protect her against the threat of revolutionary politics. The homogeneity demanded by the law and the censorship networks that police the literary text find in the Young-Girl a moral justification: the Young-Girl and the specific form of innocent enjoyment she represents function as a receptacle for a collective identity of the polis. What exactly the imagined Young-Girl is, what she thinks, what she needs and how she reads, never made explicit. This indeterminacy does not weaken the ideological power of this trope, but rather allows it to function within numerous disciplinary discourses as a moral foundation:

> The Young-Girl manages to live with a dozen unarticulated concepts, as her only philosophy, that immediately become moral categories, meaning that the whole of her vocabulary can be definitively broken down to the Good/Evil binary. It goes without saying that, in order to consider the world, it must be sufficiently simplified, and in order to permit her to live in it happily, the world must make many martyrs, starting with herself'.[15]

Throughout the trial, the Young-Girl is continually called forth as an ideal reader for the Hicklin test in order to imagine whether or not she would be corrupted and depraved by reading *Nausicaa*. The excessive investment in the figure of the Young-Girl within the trial, a trial conducted solely between men, would seem to indicate a supreme libidinal investment in this figure by the men involved. Heap was particularly canny to this investment. In 'Art and the Law', she astutely observes that:

> The society for which Mr. Sumner is agent [...] was founded to protect the public from corruption. When asked what public? Its defenders spring to the rock on which America was founded: the cream-puff of sentimentality, and answer chivalrously "Our young girls." So the mind of the young girl rules this country? In it rests the safety, progress and lustre of a nation.[16]

Heap alludes to the ironic reversal that takes place: that the Young-Girl is, in effect, ruling the nation as a sovereign, thus suggesting to a hidden, obscene aspect of the Young-Girl that both the trial and Joyce's text also suggest. The Young-Girl appears, then, to be the fantasmatic foundation upon which nation and sexual identity is founded, any interrogation of which could jeopardize the integrity of those identities.

Heap's allusion to chivalry also alludes to the tradition of courtly love. The libidinal structure of courtly love is discussed by Slavoj Žižek in his essay 'Courtly Love, or Woman as Thing'. According to Žižek, following on from Lacan, the tradition of courtly love arises from the failure of the sexual relation, the perception of the male of the traumatic Real of sexual difference. The 'Lady of Courtly Love' is originally perceived as monstrous and obscene, a radical Other who is utterly incommensurable with his desire. This radical otherness is what Lacan refers to as 'the Thing'.[17] The practices of courtly love, Žižek contends, are a response to this realization: 'The idealization of the Lady, her elevation to the spiritual, ethereal ideal, is therefore to be conceived of as [...] narcissistic projection whose function is to render her traumatic dimension invisible'.[18] The process is narcissistic in that it bestows upon the male an Imaginary identity in relation to the object cause of desire. This identity, and its concomitant enjoyment, is predicated upon never realizing the sexual union with the Lady: a continual deference and deferral is then required. What is at play in this process is the Lacanian definition of sublimation. This renunciation of desire paradoxically leads, by virtue of the continual circling around the *object a*, to a cultivation of the *jouissance* of the drive in the form of phallic *jouissance*. This process is entirely parasitic and depends upon the abjection and exclusion of the feminine from the very outset and the positing of ~~The~~ Woman in her place, with the Young-Girl being but one iteration of this fantasy figure around which the subject's desire can circulate. It is also, following on from Chu's analysis, discussed earlier a means by which the male subject rejects his own femininity by constructing the fantasy of his own masculine difference.

Both prosecution and defence posit the Young-Girl as the fictional witness at the centre of their case. The act of censorship done in order to protect the Young-Girl repeats the libidinal structure of courtly love. It is not until the world is made safe for the Young-Girl that she can be attained, but she will never be attained because she is always already threatened by corruption. Censorship in this case functions as an act of love, in the Lacanian sense, upon which identity can be founded within the Imaginary Order. American national identity, heteronormative, White and male, is thus founded upon this process.

In order to sustain this Imaginary function, the Young-Girl must also be operative at the level of the Symbolic. The figure appears in the Symbolic as a subject position to which female bodies are demanded by the big Other to conform to. We must be wary, however, to distinguish between the symbolic figure of the Young-Girl, the technique of power used to pacify resistance to biopolitics and the lived experiences of actual women. This distinction is not easy to maintain, however, and I believe that this is a symptom of the theoretical framework of Tiqqun's enquiry. Tiqqun, following a Foucauldian paradigm, suggests that the subject appears as an effect of power. Power functions through discourse so that the subject is produced at the intersection of a plurality of disciplinary discourses. This methodology makes it difficult to distinguish between the subject position determined by discourse and the subject themselves, their lived experiences are then always determined by their discursive reality, namely their designated position within the Symbolic Order. In the case of the Young-Girl, following Tiqqun's position, the women whose bodies have been coded by that discourse cannot be distinguished from the discursive figure and consequently can be interpreted as complicit with the discourse's effects of control. But the vital Lacanian intervention here is to emphasize the degree to which a subject's interpolation by discourse produces faults, lapses and symptoms that attest to the failure of this process to completely code a given subject. Copjec surmises the Foucauldian argument as 'ultimately resistant to resistance' and 'unable to conceive of a discourse that would refuse rather than refuel power'.[19] What is lacking in the panoptic schema is an appreciation for the constitutive lack within the Symbolic itself, the Real that is always missed in any act of representation. As Copjec surmises:

> The effect of representation [upon the subject] is the suspicion that some reality is being camouflaged, that we are being deceived as to the exact nature of something in itself that lies behind representation. In response to such a representation, against such a background of deception, the subject's own being breaks up between its unconscious being and its conscious semblance. At war both with its world and with itself, the subject becomes guilty of the very deceit it suspects.[20]

The subject perceives something beyond their discursive position, that something more is the Real that can never be represented. The subject then is not the effect of a multitude of disciplinary discourses, although these discourses do effect behaviours. The subject is the very excess that always already refuses all symbolic mandates from the big Other.

The consequence of both the Imaginary and Symbolic function of the Young-Girl is the continual repression and re-emergence of the Real of the Young-Girl. What is repressed in the trial is two-fold: first, no actual woman is allowed to be part of the production of a definition of the Young-Girl, most notably, in this trial, Heap and Anderson are silenced by John Quinn, their defence attorney.

But, also, the young woman who read the offending article was not allowed to be present; instead, she was represented by the prosecution and the three Judges. We have then the dimension of the Real which is the necessary resistance that any subject positioned upon the feminine side of Lacan's graph attests to, their inability to fulfil the fantasmatic demands of male desire: Women, by virtue of being subjects, are incapable of fulfilling the symbolic mandate of ~~The~~ Woman. Their silencing is thus a necessary procedure for any production of a definition of the Young-Girl that provides narcissistic access to *jouissance* for the male subject. Perhaps, this is what Heap had in mind when she argues that 'If there is anything I really fear it is the mind of the young girl'.[21] But also, perhaps, there is a more radical element towards which Heap alludes. If we conceive of the function of the Young-Girl as a fantasmatic attempt to repress the Real of sexual difference, then, perhaps, we can conceive of the trial as the site where the literary text elicits the return of the traumatic kernel at the core of the symbolic itself. We can view within the discourse of the trial a thoroughly unsuccessful attempt to define the Young-Girl through language and, in doing so, reveals the excessive amount of ideological work the Young-Girl is forced to do in the name of phallic *jouissance.* The fantasy of the Young-Girl, supposedly innocent, is traversed, and the figure is shown to be permeated with enjoyment, this is the obscene dimension of the Young-Girl, obscene in the sense that this very stain of enjoyment is that which *Nausicaa* stood accused of having shown. Put simply, in Joyce's text, the reader is presented with a sexualized woman who may or may not enjoy being the object of desire for Bloom's masturbation. Gerty Macdowell's behaviour is at odds with the fantasized purity of the figure of the Young-Girl as it appears in the discourse of the trial and the discourse of anti-obscenity. Joyce's fictional young girl is at odds with the fiction of the Young-Girl. So, in order to protect the libidinal treasure upon which their enjoyment is predicated, an enjoyment predicated on the fantasy not being understood as fantasy, the obscene double must be supressed, all female voices must be repressed to protect the fantasy of the Young-Girl.

Under Sumner's advice, Forrester decided to prosecute those responsible for the publication and sale of the July–August edition of *The Little Review.* On 29 September 1920, the NYSSV obtained copies of the July–August edition from Josephine Bell Arens, co-owner of the Washington Square Book Shop. Sumner then submitted these copies and a written complaint to Jefferson Market Police Court. The acting magistrate believed that Mr Sumner's complaint justified and issued summons for Mrs Arens to appear before the court. It was at this point that Anderson and Heap procured the services of John Quinn. Quinn, as well as a lawyer, was a collector of artworks, a patron to many modernist writers and a personal friend of Pound and Yeats. Initially hesitant to take the case due to his hostility towards Heap and Anderson, Quinn eventually agreed to defend *The Little Review* on the advice of Pound and an apparent fidelity to Joyce's novel, noting in his correspondence with Pound that a guilty verdict would 'damn the book as a whole'. Quinn's first act was to telephone Sumner and negotiate the substitution of Arens for Anderson and Heap, to which Sumner agreed.

The preliminary hearing for the trial, wherein a magistrate determines if there is enough evidence to proceed with prosecution, was held on 21 October. Surprisingly, the Magistrate, Joseph Corrigan, had decided not to hold Heap and Anderson solely on the grounds of Sumner's affidavit and read the offending article himself in order to decide. This afforded Quinn the opportunity to convince Corrigan that the text was not obscene within the meaning of the law and to test his lines of argumentation before the trial in earnest. Upon arriving in the court, Quinn observed the unusual makeup of the court room:

> There was Heap [sic] plus Anderson, and heaps of other Heaps and Andersons. Some goodlooking and some indifferent. The two rows of them looking like a fashionable whorehouse had been pinched and all its inmates hailed into court, with Heap in the role of the brazen madame. The stage was filled with police officers uniforms with glaring stars and buttons, women and men by twos and threes awaiting arraignment or sentence, niggers in the offing, chauffeurs awaiting hearings; pimps, prostitutes, hangers-on, and reporters- also whores, on the theory of 'Once a journalist always a whore'.

In this misogynist and racist description, Quinn clearly aligns himself with the law's desire to codify and regulate dissident femininities. Rather ironically, however, Quinn's misogyny, far more evident than the prosecution's, hidden behind the veil of chivalry, makes him unable to understand the function of the Young-Girl in the trial. Quinn's commentary also aligns unorthodox femininities with dissident sexualities and race and, in doing so, betrays the anxieties that these disparate groups bring about in the law; their presence is felt by him to be a destabilizing one. We can perhaps also perceive that the presence of these women and the case against a literary text may be evoking the perception of these scenes as farcical. Would not the presence of police officers and criminals be routine for the court? That these routine events take on a farcical aspect perhaps points towards a perception on Quinn's part of the obscene aspect of the law, that it too, like the literary text, is saturated with enjoyment.

The prosecution's line of argument remained consistent throughout both trials. Sumner's initial complaint, read at the preliminary hearing and the subsequent trial, summarized the prosecution's allegation against the text. According to Sumner, the July–August edition of *The Little Review*:

> Particularly upon pages 42, 43, 44, 46, 47, 48, 50, 51, 53, 55, 57, 59, 60, … is so obscene, lewd, lascivious, filthy, indecent, and disgusting, that a minute description of the same would be offensive to the Court and improper to be placed upon the record thereof.

The prosecution's case is simply that the offending pages conform to the statutory definition of obscenity as to be tested by the Hicklin test. Not much argumentation is required on behalf of the prosecution as they have simply to offer an interpretation of the text that says it does not sufficiently meet the criteria of performing a disciplinary function on the vulnerable Young-Girl. This fantasy figure testifies in absentia, through the mind of the male Magistrate. Also absent from the discourse of the preliminary hearing are the offending passages of *Nausicaa*. As discussed above, these strategic absences serve an ideological function that serves to strengthen the prosecution's case and determine the hermeneutic horizon of any reading of the text by the Magistrate.

Quinn had the very difficult task of not only disproving the prosecution's reading but also countering with a more plausible one that did not leave open the possibility of the prosecution's accusations. Quinn at first attempted to argue, much like Pound, that the literary text could never be obscene under the meaning of the law. He began by admitting 'that there [is] filth in literature and art, but it [is] not filth that would corrupt, but filth that would brace and deter'. The argument was that literature utilized the filthy only in order to strengthen the morals of the reader. This reading is similar to Pound's argument that 'the classics' served as the means upon which culture was possible. The problem with this approach is the literary text's openness to interpretation, and it can never remain stable enough from one reading to another to function as an ordering principle in quite the fashion that Pound and Quinn desire it to be. This defence is easily countered when another reader, Sumner, for instance, argues that the text does function in this way. The text invites both readings. Quinn wrestles with this problem during his defence, comparing Joyce to Rabelais and Swift in order to provide legitimacy for his argument that filth in literature has been canonized. But he also felt compelled to distinguish 'the strong hard filth of a man like Joyce with the devotion to art of a fort flabby man like Wilde'. Within Quinn's argumentation, two forms of filth are to be discerned, the phallic 'hard filth' that disciplines the reader, and the 'flabby' feminine/queer filth of writers like Wilde, which presumably would arouse in the reader some form of enjoyment in the filth depicted. The problem with this distinction is that it allows that a text defined as literary, in the case of Wilde, can also be obscene, therefore invalidating Quinn's claim that a work of literature can never be obscene. The task of discerning which representations of the abject are soft or hard remains capricious and arbitrary, the literary text does not allow for such reductive readings to remain static.

After failing to maintain his theoretical approach, Quinn changed the emphasis of his argument away from theoretical distinctions between different forms of literature and towards the text in question's effect on the reader. Quinn decided to contest the figure of the Young-Girl as the means by which obscenity should be tested. The test of obscenity should be, according to Quinn, 'its effect upon the average man or woman, not its effect upon a degenerate on one side, or a convent bred saphead on the other'. In taking this line of argument, Quinn not only departs from the precedent of the Hicklin ruling but also displays a profound ignorance for the fantasmatic function of the Young-Girl. It seems that Quinn's misogyny prevents him from adhering to the same fantasmatic dependency as the prosecution and judges in this case. For as much as Quinn traverses the fantasy of the Young-Girl, it seems that he falls into the inherent transgression of the fantasy that situates the feminine as abject but still primary. This abjection of the feminine is clearly on display when he attempts to describe a hypothetical situation in an attempt to elucidate his position:

> If a young man is in love with a woman and his mother should write to him saying: "My boy, the woman you are infatuated with is not a beautiful woman… she sweats, she stinks, she is flatulent. Her flesh is discoloured, her breath is bad. She makes ugly noises when she eats and discharges other natural functions…," those remarks might be considered by some refined person filthy, but they are not filthy within [the] meaning of the law. They would not send the aforementioned son into the arms of that fairy, but would more likely turn him from her in disgust.

Once again, the abjected female body is the site upon which the definition of male identity is founded. There is a correlation between Quinn's scenario and the encounter with the monstrous feminine described by Žižek. Quinn's analogy has literature as that with the capacity to bring about an encounter with the Other, but without the concomitant manoeuvre that sees the subject realize in the monstrous *jouissance* of the drive displayed by the Other his own enjoyment also. Instead, the male subject turns from the Other in disgust, repressing the Real of sexual difference, and retreating to the realm of fantasy. In his attempt to discredit the Young-Girl as the standard by which Joyce should be judged, Quinn has unwittingly retold the entire process by which the Young-Girl is created, so as to protect masculine identity from disintegration. But, in doing so, he has admitted literature's capacity to bring into perception the Real of sexual difference that the law has attempted to repress by its use of the Young-Girl, a figure now rendered obscene by Joyce's text and the trial. In arguing that literature forces the reader to confront this scene of absolute Otherness, albeit in the name of fortifying masculine identity, Quinn accidently acknowledges literature's capacity to destabilize the fantasmatic fabric being upheld by the law. At this moment, the very scene that Quinn expounds, and that Joyce's chapter also evokes, is being played out in the courtroom. The defence has ultimately admitted that all literature is obscene and, in doing so, has also highlighted the obscene dimension of the legal process, the fact that the law too functions as a means of regulating *jouissance* and is also stained by its presence.

Realizing the untenable nature of this line of argument, Quinn changed his position once again. In his final speech, Quinn attempted to appeal to logic. According to Quinn, neither the Young-Girl nor the average person was in danger of corruption from Joyce's text because:

> an innocent person would not understand the sex allusions and therefore could not be corrupted by them; and, for the same reason, a person who could understand them had already been "educated" and therefore could not be corrupted by them.

This defence relies on the difficulty of Joyce's text to act as a barrier to the Young-Girl. It is only those with the properly cultivated, or perhaps already corrupted, reading practices that could understand Joyce. This rhetorical ploy suffers like much of Quinn's argumentation as it admits to the openness of a text to multiple interpretations, and if any one of those could be deemed obscene within the meaning of the law, then the text could be banned. Another problem with this approach is it assumes that the Young-Girl is an actual person and not a fantasy configuration within the male psyche. The magistrate in question could read a particularly cryptic allusion to sexuality in the text and then decide that it was not appropriate for his particular Young-Girl to read.

Ultimately, this line of argumentation also failed. Corrigan upheld the Hicklin ruling and dismissed the defence that Joyce's difficulty would halt the corruption of the reader:

> There was one episode in the book that anyone could understand[...]: That was the episode where the man went off in his pants, which no one could misunderstand, and that I think is smutty, filthy within the meaning of the statue.

The problem with the text, the reason why it posed a threat to the fantasy of the Young-Girl, was not its obscurity but its readability. What Corrigan's decision indicates is a definition of obscenity that has less to do with literature embodying a threat to meaning by means of formal experimentation but rather the presence of the drive within the realm of the Symbolic Law itself, a continuous threat that requires constant policing. Quinn, upon hearing Corrigan's judgement, and remaining constant to his final argument, accused the magistrate of having 'a corrupt and depraved mind, for only a corrupt and depraved mind would understand the passage'. Corrigan and the rest of the court are said to have laughed at this accusation, and it stands as another moment of absurdity in which the law appears to acknowledge both its own inconsistency and its own knowledge of the *jouissance* upon which it depends. This uncanny moment was, however, sutured by the decision of Corrigan to hold Anderson and Heap over for trial, setting bail at $25 for each of the defendants.

The second trial, *People of the State of New York Against Margaret C Anderson and Jane Heap*, wherein it would be determined whether Heap and Anderson were guilty of publishing obscenity, took place on 14 February 1921. The case occurred in the Court of Special Sessions where the case would be presided over by three judges: Chief Justice Frederic Kernochan and Associate Justices James McInerney and Joseph Moss. Quinn made some alterations to his defence: he arranged character witnesses who would testify to the moral motives of the defendants and *The Little Review*. Quinn also arranged for witnesses to appear who would testify to Joyce's 'seriousness' and the effect of the *Nausicaa* chapter. Quinn's gambit here was the same as in the previous trial to attempt to demonstrate that the literary text can never be obscene and serves a disciplinary function. The motive in getting witnesses to testify was an attempt to show that others apart from Quinn held this view and also an attempt to predetermine the judges' readings of the text by importing reading practices from academia and psychiatry. Heap and Anderson were not to appear as witnesses and were told by Quinn to 'remain inconspicuous, meek and silent' throughout the proceedings. This tactic allowed Quinn to present the two editors as conforming to the fantasy figure of Woman, making it easier to argue that the literary work was not obscene. In practice, however, it is yet another instance of the removing any woman's voice from the debate surrounding women's sexuality. The fantasy of the Young-Girl is once again the only witness that the law can countenance.

Sumner repeated his complaint from the preliminary hearing. And Quinn began by describing who James Joyce was, listed his works, and explained his status as a serious writer of literature. These judges were not receptive to this appeal to authorial intention and responded to Quinn's introduction by asking 'what bearing those facts [had] on the subject'. The only function of the trial was, according to them, 'whether certain passages of *Ulysses* violated the statute'. Following Hicklin, the figure of the author could not be used to anchor the meaning of the text. As such, whatever Joyce's intentions were had no bearing on the effect of the text upon the reader. When this reader was the Young-Girl inside these three judges, the text would be liable for whatever the judges would read into it. Quinn, finding the judges more recalcitrant than Corrigan had been reverted to the line of argumentation that he had previously espoused, that *Ulysses* 'could not and would not corrupt people' due to its incomprehensibility. To help prove this thesis, he asked the Court to allow the testimony of expert witnesses to attest to the probable effect of the text. His request was granted, and his first witness was John Cowper Powys, an English lecturer. Powys confirmed Quinn's argument that *Ulysses*, was 'too obscure and philosophical a work to be in any sense corrupting [to the]... minds of young girls'. The second witness was Phillip Moeller of the Theatre Guild who proclaimed a similar view. Moeller began by referencing, somewhat clumsily, the discourse of psychoanalysis: *Nausicaa* was, Moeller argued, 'an unveiling of the subconscious mind in the Freudian manner', the revelations of which would have no possibility of being 'aphrodisiac in their influence'. One of the Judges at this point chastised Moeller for his recourse to Freud, Moeller was told 'you might as well talk Russian. Speak plain English if you want us to understand what you're saying'. The judges' absolute refusal to countenance any other discourse than the 'plain English' of the law demonstrates an absolute refusal to enter into any form of reciprocal relationship with the literary text. The effect of this profound obstinacy is that no meaning is produced within the trial, and it consists of separate discourses refusing to intersect. This tactic on the part of the law avoids the scenes of the previous trial where Corrigan's receptiveness to literary discourse allows the disclosure of the obscene enjoyment in the legal process. But what it does produce is an increased awareness of the law as one among a plurality of discourses, none of which operates as the means to truth, adhering to the Lacanian maxim that 'there is no metalanguage'.[22] Perhaps, to stop an awareness of this fact, Quinn was denied his wish for more witnesses. The three judges decided that the three of them would read the offending article and adjourned the trial until 21 February.

Upon recommencement, Quinn once again began a defence of the text. His speech is an amalgamation of all of his previous arguments, some of which were intensified. He emphasized the unreadability of Joyce's text by comparing it to 'a cubist painting, experimental, tentative, revolutionary, if you like, but certainly not depraving or corrupting'. He then pushed this line of argumentation further by insisting that Joyce's text was an artistic failure, a failure he claimed was due to Joyce's failing eyesight and incorrect punctuation. He finished this portion of his defence by adding 'I myself do not understand *Ulysses*, I think Joyce has carried his experiment too far in this experiment'. He then returned, somewhat contradictorily, to his former theme, that if *Ulysses* could be understood, its sexual depictions would cause disgust and not arousal. *Ulysses* was 'disgusting in portions perhaps, but no more so that Swift, Rabelais, Shakespeare, the Bible'. And, in conclusion, the text was 'neither written for nor read by school girls'. What is strange about these arguments is that they do not argue points of law or engage with the facts of the case. Whether or not Joyce intended the text to be read by young women is irrelevant, all that matters is that the text *could* be read by a woman, which it had been. Quinn's argument that the text be considered within the context of canonical writers or other artistic movements is also rendered irrelevant due to the law's interest in the effect of the text upon the Young-Girl. As for the new argument that the text is a failure and thus is impossible to read, this too is destined to fail if the prosecution can produce a reading. The openness of the text to interpretation means that foreclosing any and all readings remains impossible.

The prosecution's response was simply to read out loud the offending passages. In doing so, they could prove that the text did indeed have some meaning and that that meaning was sexual. Before reading the passage, one of the judges initially refused the prosecution permission because of Anderson's presence. After Quinn informed the Court that she was the publisher, the judge responded, 'I am sure she didn't know the significance of what she was publishing'. This is yet another example of the annexing of the feminine so as to define it between men. Eventually, she was allowed to remain, and the prosecution read the passages aloud to the court. After reading the passages, Forrester denounced *The Little Review*, Quinn, and pressed for a custodial sentence for Anderson and Heap.

> After Forrester's was completed Quinn arose and declared:
>
> If your Honors please, I offer Mr. Forrester as the defendants' chief exhibit. Just look at him, still gasping for breath at the conclusion of his denunciation, his face distorted with rage, his whole aspect apoplectic. is he filled with lewd desires? Does a reading of that chapter want to send him into the arms of a whore? Is he filled with sexual desire? Not at all. He wants to murder somebody. He wants to send Joyce to jail. He wants to send these two women to prison. He would like to disbar me. He is full of

> hatred, venom, anger, and uncharitableness. But lust? There is not a drop of lust or an ounce of sex passion in his whole body. He is filled with anger and hate. He is my chief exhibit as to the effect of *Ulysses*.

Quinn demonstrates that the effect of Ulysses is disgust, and it is an effective rhetorical manoeuvre and one that caused the judges to laugh. However, for our purposes, I wish to emphasize the degree to which disgust is itself a form of fascination. The literary text elicits this response from the prosecution, and it is in this response, in all its excessive zeal, that we can see at play another hidden aspect of the law. A sadistic will-to-punish that is itself a source of *jouissance* and one that the law must disavow. The literary text, under examination by the law, has once again elicited an encounter with the Real of enjoyment, and like in the other instances, the result has been laughter.

Quinn believed that he had sufficiently influenced the judges with this final flourish. He nearly did, with two judges deciding that they could not understand the text sufficiently to pass judgement. However, the prosecution had relied on the fact that the openness of the literary text to interpretation, even one that was a difficult as Joyce's, meant that one person could always force a reading upon it. Chief Justice Frederic Kernochan claimed that he understood the chapter and convinced the other judges of his reading. As such, the editors of *The Little Review* were found guilty of publishing obscenity, fined $50 each, and enjoined from publishing any further instalments of *Ulysses*.

Quinn's argument that *Ulysses* was unreadable ultimately failed. His argument failed for two reasons: first, his misogyny causes him to underestimate the libidinal investments in the Young-Girl within the cultural Imaginary at large. Second, the text itself betrays any single reading, even one that says that there is nothing to be read. It is this destabilizing effect of the text in relationship to the law that the trials display. This destabilizing effect is not one that appears from outside the Symbolic but rather one that is already inside the Symbolic itself. I believe that this is an aspect of many of the obscenity trials of the 20th century that critics have neglected. For instance, Parkes argues that the obscenity of Joyce's text lies in the fact that he displays forms of sexuality that are non-reproductive; by reproductive, he means both sexual reproduction but also forms and discourses of sexuality that reproduce power, the technologies of gender that require constant performativity to reproduce their effects. Joyce's transgression, for Parkes, is the 'rewriting [of] the regulatory fictions of gender and sexual identity'.[23] This rewriting has political ramifications as, through the act of rewriting, which is also an act of erasing what has come before, 'it is possible to resist the censorship of personal freedom and intellectual possibility that such fictions imply'.[24] In terms of the trial, Parkes links the formal practices of modernism with the transgression of the law that *Ulysses* stood accused:

> one of the more obviously political aspects of the text is inseparable from its function as avant-garde art, an art that disrupts and deregulates previously accepted forms of expression by refocusing our attention on the act

> of reading itself. Claiming to find "*Nausicaa*" unintelligible, the judges at the 1921 trial were responding to *Ulysses* as an obscure literary experiment. Yet their condemnation of the work as obscene implied not only that they failed to comprehend the episode, but also that its content directed attention beyond the limits of sanctioned discourse.[25]

According to this line of argument, the experimental nature of Joyce's text leads the reader's attention away from the mimetic content and towards the reader's own implication within the production of that content as a representation of reality. In doing so, the reader is forced to confront the arbitrary nature of the sanctioned discourse, that is, the realization that what appears to be natural is only so because it is sanctioned by the law, and their own complicity within that process of sanctioning and policing. But what is missed in Parkes' reading is an awareness that the content of the chapter itself is written in the same sanctioned discourse that it is deemed to transgress. *Nausicaa* is written, the first half in particular, in the style of 19th-century romance novels written for young women. It is this very investment and attention to the sanctioned discourse as discourse that begins to unravel the fantasmatic fabric it upholds. What is found to be incomprehensible by the judges is the discourse which they themselves uphold, and in this encounter with the unnameable, an obscene presence is perceived.

Parkes' accusation that the judges misread the text is also particularly telling. It positions the critic, in this case, Parkes himself, as having access to the text's truth, a truth that the judges have misunderstood. In doing so, Parkes is engaged in an act of sanctioning, endorsing the truth of the literary text, whilst simultaneously arguing that the sanctioning of the law is arbitrary and ignorant. In contrast, I wish to argue that we are not dealing with a misreading of the text's truth, one which I have access to. Instead, I wish to argue that the judges perceived a truth inaccessible to that of the literary critic. It was not that the judges read the text incorrectly, but that their position as arbitrators of the sanctioned discourse allowed them to perceive the text in a way incommensurable to the critic.

In this trial, the critic has been positioned as the defender of the text's value against the accusations of the law: a voice that is continually silenced by the law. Future changes in the law would allow for an increased value to be placed upon experts in literary studies to prove that the literary text had value to society at large. As such, these very tensions between the critic and the text's truth and the structural similarities between the law and literary criticism as discourses of truth would be worked through in the re-trial of *Ulysses* that took place in 1933.

Notes

1 The 1873 Act for the "Suppression of Trade in, and Circulation of, Obscene Literature and Articles of Immoral Use", known colloquially as the Comstock Laws, after its instigator Anthony Comstock, criminalized the use of the U.S. Postal Service for the distribution of obscene materials. These included:

> an obscene book, pamphlet, paper, writing, advertisement, circular, print, picture, drawing or other representation, figure, or image on or of paper or other

> material, or any cast instrument, or other article of an immoral nature, or any drug or medicine, or any article whatever, for the prevention of conception, or for causing unlawful abortion.
>
> (Section 211 of the United States Criminal Code)

The penalty for such action was a maximum prison sentence of five years or a fine ranging between 100 and 2000 dollars. Despite Pound's claims of idiocy on the part of the law makers, there is evidence in the discourse of the subsequent obscenity trials to suggest that the seemingly disparate subjects of literature, abortion and drugs, all came to embody in different ways a solipsistic *jouissance* that threatened to erode the fantasmatic basis of American national identity, and perhaps all forms of identification that the law protects.

2 Ezra Pound, 'The Classics Escape', in *The Little Review*, Vol. 5, No. 11, 1918, pp. 32–34, p. 33.
3 Quoted in Ibid. p. 34.
4 Ibid.
5 Jane Heap, 'Art and the Law', in *The Little Review*, Vol. VII, No. 3, Sep–Dec, pp. 5–7, p. 5.
6 It was the defence offered in the trial of *Madame Bovary* by Marie-Antoine-Jules Senard. Senard's argument was successful in that case, thereby setting a precedent for all subsequent defences of the literary text. This will also inform the later successful defences of both *Ulysses* and *Lady Chatterley's Lover* that I will explore in detail in Chapters 3 and 4.
7 The details of the case and all quotations from it, unless otherwise referenced, are sourced from Paul Vanderham, *James Joyce and Censorship: The Trials of "Ulysses"*, (New York: New York University Press, 1997).
8 Quoted in John Sumner, 'The Truth about "Literary Lynching"', in *The Dial*, Vol. 71, 1921, pp. 63–67, p. 66.
9 Rachel Potter, *Obscene Modernism: Literary Censorship and Experiment 1900–1940*, (Oxford: Oxford University Press, 2013), p. 36.
10 Friedrich Kittler, *Discourse Networks 1800/1900*, trans. Chris Cullens and Michael Metteer, (Stanford, CA: Stanford University Press, 1992), p. 255.
11 Initially, the society was headed by Anthony Comstock. Sumner took over as Executive Secretary in 1915, increasing the amount of legal action against suspected distributors.
12 Sumner, 'The Truth about "Literary Lynching"', p. 66.
13 Ibid. p. 77.
14 Tiqqun, *Preliminary Materials for a Theory of the Young Girl*, trans. Ariana Reines, (London: Semiotext(e), 2012), p. 15.
15 Ibid. p. 26. For the purpose of clarity, I shall, using Tiqqun's parlance, distinguish between the symbolic figure of the Young-Girl by capitalizing and hyphenating the term, the female subjects whom this term attempts to define will be referred to without capitalization and hyphenation, that is, young girls.
16 Heap, 'Art and the Law', p. 5.
17 Jacques Lacan, *Seminar VII: The Ethics of Psychoanalysis*, trans. Dennis Porter, (London: Routledge, 1992), p. 9.
18 Slavoj Žižek, 'Courtly Love or Woman as Thing', in *The Žižek Reader*, ed. Elizabeth Wright and Edmond Wright, (London: Blackwell Publishing, 1999), pp. 148–173, p. 151.
19 Joan Copjec, *Read My Desire*, (London: MIT Press, 1994), p. 33.
20 Ibid. pp. 37–38.
21 Heap, 'Art and the Law', p. 6.
22 Lacan, *Seminar XX*, p. 118.
23 Parkes, *Theater*, p. 68.
24 Ibid.
25 Ibid.

Bibliography

Copjec, Joan, *Read My Desire*, (London: MIT Press, 1994).

Heap, Jane, 'Art and the Law', in *The Little Review*, Vol. VII, No. 3, Sep–Dec 1920, pp. 5–7.

Kittler, Friedrich, *Discourse Networks1800/1900*, trans. Chris Cullens and Michael Metteer, (Stanford, CA: Stanford University Press, 1992).

Lacan, Jacques, *Seminar VII: The Ethics of Psychoanalysis*, trans. Dennis Porter, (London: Routledge, 1992).

———, *Seminar XX: On Feminine Sexuality: The Limits of Love and Knowledge*, trans. Bruce Fink, (London: Norton, 1999).

Potter, Rachel, *Obscene Modernism: Literary Censorship and Experiment 1900–1940*, (Oxford: Oxford University Press, 2013).

Pound, Ezra, 'The Classics Escape', in *The Little Review*, Vol. 5, No. 11, 1918, pp. 32–34.

Sumner, John, 'The Truth about "Literary Lynching"', in *The Dial*, Vol. 71, 1921, pp. 63–67.

Tiqqun, *Preliminary Materials for a Theory of the Young Girl*, trans. Ariana Reines, (London: Semiotext(e), 2012).

Vanderham, Paul, *James Joyce and Censorship: The Trials of "Ulysses"*, (New York: New York University Press, 1997).

Žižek, Slavoj, 'Courtly Love or Woman as Thing', in *The Žižek Reader*, ed. Elizabeth Wright and Edmond Wright, (London: Blackwell Publishing, 1999), pp. 148–173.

PART 2

~~The~~ Truth

Father can't you see, I'm writing!

During the course of these trials, the literary text is caught between two truth claims: It is the dangerous corrupting substance, moving the subject away from truth or it is the means by which truth is attained, a supplement that allows the subject access to a form of truth that was previously obscured. It is then either a dangerous simulacrum of the truth or the means by which the truth and the simulacrum are to be distinguished. The point of this thesis is not to argue for one or the other truth claim's legitimacy but rather to posit that both claims to the truth of the text are dependent on forms of work, modes of reading and the repression of aspects of the text heterogeneous to the respective claim. In short, the truth of the text is undecidable, and the legal decision does not consist in the evaluation of the text's essence but rather in the act of naming a particular truth claim legitimate and the other illegitimate. The need for decision attests to what Dennis Schep refers to as an 'addiction to truth' locatable in both sides of this binary.[1] So, the question the following chapters attempt to answer is not how the truth of *Ulysses* and *Lady Chatterley's Lover* was discovered and legitimated by the law, but rather how were these novels' relationships with that category produced, what labour was required and what investments motivated this translation of *Ulysses* from pornography to literature.

To further explore this connection between the literary text, truth, the undecidable, the law and the discourse of drugs, I will call upon Jacques Derrida and others' work on the concept of the *pharmakon*. After delineating the theoretical foundations of my enquiry, this chapter will explore the parallels between the literary text and intoxicating substances in philosophy and in obscenity trials

DOI: 10.4324/9781003202509-2

arguing that the legal responses to both writing considered obscene and drugs considered dangerous constitute a pharmacological management of the subject and her enjoyment. The trial will then be analysed as a space in which the production of a new pharmacology of the literary text emerges alongside the production of a new fantasy formation that replaces the Young-Girl as the normative reader, the *homme moyen sensual.*

In his essay 'Plato's Pharmacy', Derrida explores the fundamental ambiguity of the Greek term *pharmakon* and its derivatives. Commenting on Plato's *Phaedrus*, Derrida focuses on Socrates's definition of the writing as a *pharmakon*, the Greek term for both poison and cure. The written signifier, for Socrates, is not neutral, and it is thus the duty of the philosopher to ask 'the question of propriety and impropriety in writing' and to set out 'the conditions which make it proper or improper'.[2] This analysis originates in the problem posed by the act of speech writing, wherein the speaker is not concomitant with the author, and thus the subject speaks words that are not his own. Writing thus comes to be associated with absence, whilst 'living speech' retains the presence of the *logos*, the presence of meaning. Writing comes to represent a split between the subject and his words, an orphaning of the word from its father.

To elucidate further on this distinction between living speech as the locus of truth and the dead letter as the harbinger of falsehood, Socrates relates a myth to Phaedrus on the origin of writing.[3] Socrates tells the story of the Egyptian god Theuth and his attempt to offer King Thamus the gift of writing. The written signifier would allow the truth to remain present in the absence of the subject who first enunciated it: 'My discovery' Theuth states, 'provides a recipe (*pharmakon*) for memory and wisdom'.[4] Writing is presented as a *pharmakon*, here a beneficial supplement to the spoken word, the guarantor of its meaning. However, Thamus sees in the written signifier a threat to the logos it is supposed to protect:

> If men learn this, it will implant forgetfulness in their souls: they will cease to exercise memory because they rely on that which is written, calling things to remembrance no longer from within themselves, but by means of external marks.[5]

The sovereign perceives that the advent of writing would have the opposite effect from the one originally devised: a corrosion of the logos. Key to this analysis are two anxieties, one concerning the collapse of the boundary between the inside and outside and the other a dependency that the subject would develop towards the signifier: the emergence of the *pharmakon* raises the question of addiction. What is both saved and initiated in the sovereign's decision to exclude writing is the distinction between interior and exterior. Addiction presupposes the dependency of the subject upon an exterior object thus reversing the previous privileging of interiority: in addiction, the other takes precedence over the subject.

There are also political consequences to this refusal: According to the king, 'it is no true wisdom that you offer your disciples, but only its semblance; [...]

and as men filled, not with wisdom but with the conceit of wisdom, they will be a burden to their fellows'.[6] The inability to distinguish between truth and semblance, and the potential addiction towards the latter, creates in the addicted subject a further dependency upon his fellow citizens who choose the path of truth. According to this view, a cohesive society requires a shared conception of the truth and a means by which it can be distinguished from falsehood. This distinction takes place in the form of the law and the figure of the sovereign who decides upon truth and fiction for his subjects. What is evaded in the sovereign's response is the fact that, by virtue of the introduction of a remedy, an initial problem inherent within the logos requires the intervention of the *pharmakon* in the first place. To admit the *pharmakon* would be to undermine the sovereign's self-sufficiency and render the decision by which the *pharmakon* is both distinguished and excluded arbitrary. In this way, the sovereign, too, can be conceived as an addict. Addicted to truth, the sovereign is dependent upon the act of decision itself and thus upon the *pharmakon* whose emergence both demands censure and troubles the foundations upon which the decision to exclude it is legitimated.

After telling Phaedrus this myth of the creation of writing, Socrates goes on to describe in more detail the deficiencies of the written word as compared to speech. The problem with written letters, argues Socrates, is that

> [t]hey seem to talk to you as though they were intelligent, but if you ask them anything about what they say, from a desire to be instructed, they go on telling you the same thing for ever. And once a thing is put in writing [...] [it] drifts all over the place, getting into the hands, not only of those who understand it, but equally those who have no business with it; it doesn't know how to address the right people, and not address the wrong. And when it is ill-treated and unfairly abused it always needs it parent to come to its help being unable to defend or help itself.[7]

Socrates's suspicion of the written word is contradictory: words' inability to speak more than they signify denotes an inherent lack but the written word also says too much to too many people. When divorced from the speaking subject the signifier is both independent and powerful whilst also being, at the same time, impotent and requiring assistance. The power, and thus the danger, of the written words is their ability to 'drift', that is, their capacity for a free dissemination that transgresses boundaries. The written word functions here as the double of the sovereign in that it constitutes an exception to the laws and distinctions operative within the community. The anxiety operative throughout this passage is the inability to police the signifier's destination and its interpretation once it arrives: Meaning cannot be maintained and the knowledge that these signifiers are supposed to represent cannot be said to be true. However, the written word is also characterized as a child 'unable to defend or help itself' and requiring parental intervention.

A double supplementation of the original analysis is required for the signifier to lose its power. First, a will to be understood, or rather a will to truth, is supposed on the part of the signifier itself, whereas before the absence of intention, the dead repetition that was only a semblance of life had been the source of Socrates's suspicion. The signifier begins this passage as the vehicle for a carefree enjoyment in the act of repetition that threatens society and then shifts into a state of victimhood desiring the intervention of some other agent. Second, the father, the sovereign and the law are the means by which the signifier and the truth they now wish to signify are saved. The result of the addition of these two supplements is the transformation of the signifier from the sovereign's destructive double into the sovereign's child and from the meaningless destructive *jouissance* to a desire to be put into use for the good of the community.

Derrida, in his reading of Plato's text, discerns this fundamental ambiguity operative within Socrates's ambivalence towards the written word. The emergence of the *pharmakon* necessitates the creation of a space in which a decision must be made and adulteration, regulation and management strategies must be put in place to prevent the emergence once again: that place, Derrida argues, is the pharmacy. As Derrida states:

> [i]n the pharmacy [one cannot] distinguish the medicine from the poison, the good from the evil, the true from the false, the inside from the outside, the vital from the mortal, the first from the second, etc. Conceived within this original reversibility, the *pharmakon* is the same precisely because it has no identity.[8]

The pharmacy is then the zone in which the foundations of the law, the claims to truth upon which it functions, are legitimated by the violent suppression of the *pharmakon*. But, in this violent act, those truths are shown to depend upon the intervention of violence, undermining their assumed self-sufficiency. The pharmacy is then a lawless space, a state of exception where the only form of control is violence. The law is then marked by a dependency on, an addiction to, the *pharmakon*. This dependency is evidenced in the numerous symptoms, or coping mechanisms, of the law such as the prohibition and management of the *pharmakon* itself. The taxonomy and regulation of potentially threatening substances, written or otherwise, constitutes the law's response to the challenge to its own legitimacy by the *pharmakon*. Commenting on the law's compulsion to understand the *pharmakon*, the law's will to truth, Dennis Schep argues that 'clear demarcations cover up the *pharmakon*'s elusive threat / threatening elusiveness, hiding legislative logic's blind leap into being and its absence of exterior foundations under a veil of clear-cut categories with a semblance of durability'.[9] The law demands that the *pharmakon* present itself as it truly is, to which the *pharmakon* cannot comply. This inability to be brought within the inside of the law challenges the power of the law to designate boundaries and identities. A decision is thus taken by the law, a split is enacted in the *pharmakon*, and the untranslatable is translated into two separate categories: inside/outside, good/evil, medicine/drug and literature/obscenity.

But, in this act of translation, the sovereign decision upon the undecidable, a trace remains of that schism. Commenting on the subsequent translations of Plato's dialogue and of the word *pharmakon* itself into poison or remedy, Derrida comments that:

> [a]ll translations [of Plato's Phaedrus] into languages that are the heirs and depositaries of Western metaphysics thus produce on the *pharmakon* an effect of analysis that violently destroys it, reduces it to one of its simple elements by interpreting it, paradoxically enough, in the light of the ulterior developments it itself has made possible. Such an interpretative translation is thus as violent as it is impotent: it destroys the *pharmakon* but at the same time forbids itself access to it, leaving it untouched in its reserve.[10]

To translate *pharmakon* into a singular word, or, in another register, to subject being to the Symbolic order, necessitates the repression of all that within the *pharmakon* that cannot be contained within that decision. The decision, although it must appear final, leaves traces, or symptoms, of those repressed aspects, testifying to the untenable nature of the legal decision and its dependency upon that which it has expelled. One of these traces can be seen in Socrates's categorization of the written word and its distinction from speech. Here, it is the signifier itself that functions as the *pharmakon*, demanding a distinction between speech and writing, wherein, with the help of numerous supplements, speech is privileged as the vehicle for life and being and truth and writing is designated as the place of death, falsehood and non-being. But, even after this, split has taken place, and a further split has taken place within the written word: it is all powerful but also impotent. This ambiguity testifies to an instability operative within speech itself, and thus, within the very decision to split the signifier into these categories.

This understanding of law's relation to the *pharmakon* allows us to conceptualize the space of the obscenity trial as a form of pharmacy, wherein the law's relation to itself as language is brought to the fore. In the previous two chapters, I have explored the ways in which the obscene literary text was designated by the law as the means by which untruth, death and dissident sexuality were disseminated throughout society. In doing so, the law made a clear distinction between its own function and that of obscenity. The law was on the side of order, community, health and the sexual relation, and the obscene text became the place holder for all the antimonies of these virtues.[11] But in the two trials that follow, the texts are presented not as dangerous drugs but rather as beneficial texts for the public, a stimulus for positive and healthy enjoyment rather than the destructive *jouissance* they had previously been accused of harbouring. I will argue that it is the discourse of literary criticism that helps enact this translation from poison to remedy. In a sense, the literary critic has a pharmacological function: upon encountering the undecidable within the literary text, the critic then decides to translate what he finds into a claim to truth. The critic, like the law, is driven by a will, or addiction, to truth.[12]

Notes

1 Dennis Schep, *Drugs: Rhetoric of Fantasy, Addiction to Truth*, (Dresden: Atropos Press, 2011), p. 6.
2 Plato, *Phaedrus*, trans. Reginald Hackforth, (Cambridge: Cambridge University Press, 1997), p. 156.
3 In the face of the undecidable distinction between the dead letter and living speech, Socrates introduces a myth of a time before the advent of writing, before the law. The law that governs the exclusion of the written word into the Real of untruth is itself founded upon a fiction and is thus dependent upon that which it feels compelled to exclude. The truth in the name of which Socrates denounces writing is itself based upon 'a rumour', that which has been repeated by others. The dead letters of these presumably dead others speak through Socrates at this point, if only to then exclude themselves in the sovereign decision of Theuth.
4 Ibid. p. 157.
5 Ibid. p. 137.
6 Ibid. p. 157.
7 Ibid. p. 159.
8 Jacques Derrida, *Dissemination*, trans. Barabara Johnson, (London: Athlone, 1981), p. 31.
9 Schep, *Drugs*, p. 19.
10 Derrida, *Dissemination*, p. 36.
11 And perhaps in the split between the 'good' literary text and the 'bad' obscene text is the trace of a previous decision between law and literature in which the law renounces its own status as writing. If this is the case, the operation of obscenity is the means by which the law continues to deny its own status as writing by giving itself the responsibility to police that which it has defined as its opposite.
12 Again, the problem of the addict opens up the pharmacological dimension of desire: the will would seem to imply a form of desire based within the subject that moves outwards into the world into the dimension of the other. In contrast, the addicted subject's will is not his own, the object of the addiction is given precedence and the subject's desire is founded not in themselves but in the dimension of the other.

Bibliography

Derrida, Jacques, *Dissemination*, trans. Barabara Johnson, (London: Athlone, 1981).
Plato, *Phaedrus*, trans. Reginald Hackforth, (Cambridge: Cambridge University Press, 1997).
Schep, Dennis, *Drugs: Rhetoric of Fantasy, Addiction to Truth*, (Dresden: Atropos Press, 2011).

3

WOOLSEY'S PHARMACY

On 5 December 1933, The United States Government ratified the Twenty-First Amendment to the United States Constitution. The amendment repealed the Eighteenth Amendment that had prohibited the 'transportation or importation into any State, Territory, or possession of the United States for delivery or use therein of intoxicating liquors'.[1] The next day, 6 December, Judge John M. Woolsey declared *Ulysses* not obscene under the legal definition of that word thus allowing Random House to publish Joyce's text and reversing the 1922 decision that condemned the text as obscene. As of this date, Americans were free to sell, purchase and enjoy articles and substances that were previously coded by the law as corrupting bodies, morals, the family and the sexual health of the nation.

The concurrence of these two events in legal history would at first seem coincidental. Both were products of separate campaigns and individuals working within very different legal contexts: the laws that circumscribe the dissemination of texts are very different from those that delineate and restrict the movement of intoxicating substances. However, Woolsey's decision contains numerous references to alcohol and other drugs: *Ulysses* is a 'rather strong draught' and 'emetic' in effect but is judged not obscene by virtue of the fact that 'nowhere does it tend to be an aphrodisiac'.[2] In comparing the effect of literature to drugs, Woolsey is both implying a correspondence between the intoxicating effects of drugs and literature as well as demarcating the acceptable effects of these substances and the deleterious ones: the emetic is acceptable and the aphrodisiac is coded as obscene. Woolsey's dependency upon the discourse of drugs in order to legitimate *Ulysses* attests to a wider cultural moment in which America was restructuring its relation to intoxication in its many forms. However, this dependency points towards the difficulty in organizing a stable position in relation to intoxication itself: Woolsey requires the perceived stable distinction between good drugs and bad drugs to base his judgement of the text's beneficial effects. The discourse

DOI: 10.4324/9781003202509-3

of drugs functions as a supplement upon which the presence of the text and its effects can be founded: it attests to the inability for Woolsey to base the meaning and effects of the text upon the text itself, an admission of the non-presence of the text as an object of knowledge. I intend to show, however, that the drawing of a difference between good and bad drugs takes places at the very moment in which Woolsey's own enunciation shifts to re-incorporate alcohol into the taxonomy of legitimate intoxicants.

This chapter will explore the connections, intersections and impasses that emerge when the discourses of drugs and literature engage within the courtroom. As I have shown in the previous chapters, the category of the obscene functions within a binary in which it names that which is not literature. This apparently clear split is troubled in the legal court, however. The law's need to render a decision upon the accused text problematizes rather than clarifies the distinction between literature and obscenity. The legal decision, as both *R v Methuen* and the 1922 *Little Review* trial attest, renders the division untenable. The trials attest to the undecidable distinction between the pornographic and the literary, the stain of obscenity at the core of the signifier. The literary text is that which is both too full of meaning and at the same time too lightweight to attest to its own value and presence.

The 1933 trial distinguishes itself from the previous two trials I have discussed in the way the defence of the book is based upon a range of supplementary texts prepared in advance by the legal team. These supplements, exterior to the body of the text and later fixed to it, help stabilize the meaning of *Ulysses* under the gaze of the law by placing the novel within a context of other texts and within the literary category of the classic. It is around this category that the defence argues for *Ulysses*' legitimacy. A double movement is at play here: on the one hand, *Ulysses* is a classic in that it corresponds to a pre-existing category. On the other hand, there is the demonstrable labour of the literary critics and the lawyers as to the novel's self-evident status as classic. Avital Ronell, in reference to the obscenity trials of Flaubert and Burroughs, argues that

> Literature has to be seen wearing something external to itself, it cannot simply circulate its non-being, and almost any article will do. This would affirm at least one value of the book review as that legal work which covers up the work.[3]

Ronell distinguishes between two forms of work: the work of the law and the work of the literary text. The work of the text is towards the circulation of its non-being that, which in Chapter 1, I have discussed in terms of the death drive and destructive *jouissance*. There, I discussed this form of *jouissance*'s relation to truth as an enjoyment in the absence of truth as well as the threat that this form of enjoyment poses to the truth claims of ideology. The work of the law was to censure the texts that were felt to be the catalysts for this destructive sexual force. The binary was clear in these cases, and the obscene text was on the side of non-being, non-truth and non-reproductive sexuality, whereas the law was on the side of presence, truth and heteronormativity. But, in Ronell's analysis, the book review, the work of the literary critic, attempts to translate the literary text from non-being into presence. This chapter will explore the function of literary criticism in the 1933 *Ulysses* trial, in which the literary criticism works upon the novel to produce a structured text marked by it serious artistic intent, honest representation of life and comprehensible structure all aspects which were not perceived in the 1922 trial and formed the basis for the text's censorship.

The cultural anxieties around the uses and effects of alcohol on public health and a desire to curtail or prohibit alcohol's consumption began in earnest during the latter half of the 19th century. Much like the vigilance societies formed to police obscene texts, much of the early work towards prohibition was undertaken by voluntary societies such as The Woman's Christian Temperance Union. Formed in 1874, the WCTU campaigned for the change in American attitudes to drink on religious and moral grounds, arguing that alcohol served as a sinful distraction from Christian duties as well as hindered the cause of female emancipation.[4] Their function was, according to their first President, Anne Wittenmyer, to 'replace the brandy flask in the pocket of a drinking man by the Bible'.[5] One can see here operative a logic of the supplement whereby man is marked by a lack in need of supplementation, the form of the supplement can either be divine in the case of God and his own supplement, the Bible, or evil in the case of alcohol. The evil caused by alcohol is framed as damage done to the individual and national body. In the same text, the emergence of alcohol is interpreted as destroying a previous and idyllic state, or more accurately, a potential that existed in the past and, as such, could still be recovered:

> [W]e might have been the strongest and richest nation in the world had not our rulers in their unwisdom encouraged the liquor traffic [...] which has been destructive to our moral, industrial, and financial interests. [...] The whole land was filled with beggary and crime[...] Millions who ought to have been producers and bread-winners, became consumers, tramps and criminals. Men, mad with strong drink, reeled through the streets; women, grown old before their time, toiled in their comfortless homes in dumb despair, and little half-starved children hid away in fear from their brutal fathers. It was with us as it was with the Egyptians—there was one dead in almost every house.[6]

Alcohol is figured as a divine plague that has ravaged America leading to the death and suffering of those coded as non-drinkers, women and children. Masculinity itself is put into peril by alcohol too: men themselves are caused to lose their natural masculine destiny as 'bread-winners' and 'producers' in favour of consumption, 'madness' and destruction, those very aspects of enjoyment and non-truth felt to be dangerous and embodied in both literature and the category of drugs. But we can also see here operative an aspect of the temperance movement that would have much wider reaching implications for the support of a nationwide prohibition: the financial cost of alcohol consumption, that is, the damage that intoxication bears upon production. The wealth of the nation and the health of the nation become intertwined here with the intoxicated male subject and his enjoyment being figured as destructive towards both.

And it was this rationalist line of argument that distinguished the rhetoric and strategies of the Anti-Saloon League with those of the more moralizing arguments of the WCTU. The ASL functioned in a much more focused and directly political manner aiming to change legislation first and hearts and minds later. Key to winning support was the argument that America's productivity and wealth was put at risk by alcohol consumption. Bataille, discussing the links between Protestant suspicion of alcohol and the emergence of a capitalist ethics, discusses this economic aspect of alcohol:

> alcohol, whose consumption does not enable us to work more - or even deprives us, for a time, of our strength to produce. Idleness [...] or alcohol have the advantage of consuming without a return - without a profit - the resources that they use: They simply satisfy us; they correspond to the unnecessary choice that we make of them.[7]

Alcohol disrupts an economy of mutual exchange and growth by introducing a destructive element; its consumption is defined by the absence of profit. This enjoyment without return, this surplus enjoyment, produced by alcohol was coded by the temperance movement as waste and a form of waste that left America under threat from foreign powers. In *Dry Manhattan*, Michael Lerner links the American entry into the First World War with growing support for prohibition:

> The league [...] promoted the benefits of temperance for American soldiers, arguing that sober soldiers were safer, healthier, and less likely to divulge wartime secrets. Tapping into the rapid rise of anti-German sentiment in the United States, the league also questioned the loyalty and political activities of German-American brewers, demonizing them as a threat to domestic productivity.[8]

The destructive enjoyment inherent in the consumption and effects of alcohol was not only felt as halting American growth, as a retardant, but also as a gain for the enemy. Enjoyment is thus doubled, present in the intoxicated subject in its destructive form and also within its positive utilizable form but in a form of having been taken by the German state: Germany is stealing the good enjoyment by selling the bad one, leading to a net loss for the American nation. America felt itself lacking in positive enjoyment, and alcohol was identified as the reason for this loss.

In response to this perceived loss in productivity and potential profit, American industry began to support calls for legal prohibition and put into place financial incentives and surveillance strategies in the belief that a moral worker was a productive worker. Antonio Gramsci, commenting on Henry Ford's 'Five Dollar Day' initiative, argues that the prohibition of alcohol was entirely necessary for the production of a new type of worker who would in turn be necessary for the complete rationalized form of capitalist production without waste:

> In America rationalization of work and prohibition are undoubtedly connected. The enquiries conducted by the industrialists into the workers' private lives and the inspection services created by some firms to control the 'morality' of their workers are necessities of the new methods of work. [...] a new type of worker and of man ...developing in the worker to the highest degree automatic and mechanical attitudes, breaking up the old psycho-physical nexus of qualified professional work, which demands a certain active participation of intelligence, fantasy and initiative on the part of the worker, and reducing productive operations exclusively to the mechanical, physical aspect. [...] it is a phase which will itself be superseded by the creation of a psycho-physical nexus of a new type. Both different from its predecessors and undoubtedly superior.[9]

These modes of surveillance varied in intrusiveness but were ultimately designed to change the working class's relation to their own bodies and pleasures, thus eliminating any surplus that could not be incorporated into the economy and into the production of wealth. This mechanization of the worker meant that the surplus that was being targeted was the worker's enjoyment itself, and the subject must learn to enjoy in a productive matter and must be shorn of his attachments to 'fantasy', the sexual aspect of his existence that work could not accommodate for. By stating that this new mode of subjectivity would be 'superior', Gramsci argues that this transformation of the subject's relation to work and sexuality is a necessary precondition for a future transition to communism. This transformation would lead to 'a new form of sexual union shorn of the bright and dazzling colour of the romantic tinsel typical of the petit bourgeois and Bohemian layabout'.[10] For both the capitalist Ford and the Marxist Gramsci, the consumption of alcohol functioned as a hindrance to the necessary transformation of the subject; for Ford, it was necessary for increased productivity and wealth accumulation; for Gramsci, it would be necessary to resist advertising based upon the commodity fetishism thus helping the emergence of a rational class consciousness. The *pharmakon* of alcohol then refuses a political position, refuses to be of use and as such is figured as enemy to both left and right.

This ambiguity was not just evident on the extremes of politics but all across the spectrum: alcohol and its zone of purchase, the saloon, was utilized by advocates of prohibition as a polysemic signifier that could embody any fear or anxiety that suited the cause of prohibition. Daniel Bell in *The Cultural Contradictions of Capitalism* highlights the many ways in which alcohol could be coded for political gain:

> The attack on the saloon allowed the Prohibition movement to bring together many diverse elements under one political banner. For the small-town native American Protestant, the saloon epitomized the social habits of the immigrant population. For the Progressive, the saloon was the source of the corruption he felt to be the bane of political life. For the Populist, it became the root of his antipathy to the debilitating effects of urban life.[11]

Anxieties linked to issues of race, gender and class were all mobilized in order to locate their cause in alcohol consumption: the enjoyment that the other was hoarding and that the subject felt was their own by right was offered to them by the prohibition movement.

With the help of American industry, savvy political manoeuvring from the ASL and a delayed and ineffectual opposition the prohibition of alcohol was written in to the constitution as the 18th Amendment in January 1919 and the National Prohibition Act set in place the means by which the Amendment would be enforced nationally. On 6 January 1920, America officially became a dry nation.

The effect of prohibition and literary censorship was not the end of the dissemination of useless enjoyment but rather the outsourcing of that enjoyment from America towards other nations whose laws allowed for the production and distribution of both intoxicating substances and sexually explicit texts. Rachel Potter in *Obscene Modernism* highlights the case of Obelisk Press in France as an example of a publisher who, due to the lax French censorship laws in regard to texts published in English, began to publish both texts recognized as pornography and works of purported literary merit that had been banned in English speaking countries for obscenity, most importantly Henry Miller's *Tropic of Cancer.*[12] We have here an instance of the obscene double to the reputable publisher seen in the trial of *The Rainbow*. Methuen's name signified that beyond itself which was pure and true. The obscene publicist takes on the contrary position wherein the name of Obelisk and other publishers of that ilk come to occupy a double position of both the exploitation of sex for money and high art which could transcend the accusation of exploitation by virtue of its artistic merit. It is still apparent here that it is sex that occurs as a problem here: only once mobilized in the name of art and truth can sex be redeemed of its troubling and destabilizing power, a power always linked to the market in the figure of the pornographer.

Potter's analysis is important here because it shows how this ambiguity as regards these publishers is an effect of the obscenity laws themselves not necessarily some inherent link between pornography and high modernism: by banning these works, the law thus creates the conditions for these publishers to produce these texts out of a sense of duty towards art. However, as a result of the reputation, these texts had after the law's designation of them as obscene, only publishers of pornographic texts felt comfortable publishing them, as it would not harm their reputation but only increase it as well as increasing sales. On the subject of Jack Kahane, founder of Obelisk press, Dirk Van Hulle, argues that

> publishing an avant-garde work could establish an independent publisher's reputation, even if it was not an immediate commercial success; but [...] it also worked the other way round: since Kahane was one of the few expatriate publishers in interwar Paris who could not rely on a wealthy family or partner, he could only publish avantgarde novels if he was able to make a profit from publishing so-called 'd.b.'s (dirty books) – several of them written by Kahane himself.[13]

The 'dirty books' were then funding the ambitions of the publicists rather than testifying to an essential link between pornography and high modernism. However, that link remains operative because of this necessity produced by the law which stained these texts with the suspicion of obscenity as well as foreclosing the ambitions of these publishers to one day rid themselves of the title of pornographer. It is the act of policing obscenity that produces the figure of the pornographer/publisher who maintains an ambivalent position as both sexual deviant and saviour of the arts which in turn produces a similar undecidability in the texts published by the publisher.

The presence of these publishers in France printing in English meant that American and British subjects could acquire texts that were not available in their own countries leading to an influx of obscene literature back into these nations. Knowledge of this trade led both to the association in British and American culture between obscene literature with continental Europe, in particular Paris, which in turn led to the creation of new laws designed to stem the flow of these texts into Britain and America. As I have demonstrated in previous chapters, the destructive *jouissance* for which numerous texts and substances come to signify is itself transferable but not removable from language. This thesis is an analysis of how the literary text transforms from an embodiment of this destructive enjoyment and into an object or practice of useful public good from destructive *jouissance* to meaningful desire, and because this desire is meaningful, it can be managed, reproduced and commercialized.

Prohibition and literary censorship found their justification in a need to rid the national body of this form of enjoyment which was thought to be corrupting the collective national identity and shared values of its citizens. But after legal attempts to flush out this foreign enjoyment, its foreign quality is multiplied by the fact those signifiers of foreign enjoyment returning back to American shores from areas coded as heterogeneous to that form of identity which needed to be protected: in the case of literature France, in the case of alcohol, Canada, Mexico and the nations of the Caribbean. The presence of these goods in American cities and households testified to the permeability of national boundaries and the difficulty in policing those boundaries beyond edicts of prohibition.[14]

This suspicion of foreign goods destroying American life was greatly exacerbated by the onset of the Great Depression in 1929. In response to this extreme economic slump, the United States Government passed the 1930 Tariff Act which raised tariffs on international goods in a Protectionist move aimed at securing the stability of American jobs. When the matter of policing immoral articles came to be re-written, the wording of the act is interesting for the manner in which it collects many disparate articles under that category:

> All persons are prohibited from importing into the United States from any foreign country any book, pamphlet, paper, writing, advertisement, circular, print, picture, or drawing containing any matter advocating or urging treason or insurrection against the United States, or forcible resistance to any law of the United States, or containing any threat to take the life of or inflict bodily harm upon any person in the United States, or any obscene book, pamphlet, paper, writing, advertisement, circular, print, picture, drawing, or other representation, figure, or image on or of paper or other material, or any cast, instrument, or other article which is obscene or immoral, or any drug or medicine or any article whatever for causing unlawful abortion.[15]

Just as in the Comstock Laws that were used to prosecute *The Little Review* a decade earlier, the Tariff Act condenses political sedition against the nation, representations of sexuality and contraception.[16] All three constitute forms of enjoyment that are perceived as solitary and as potentially divorcing the subject from the polis and thus threatening the very nature of that polis as a form of collective identity.

Though the same objects were declared contraband as the previous Comstock Act had stipulated, the Act however contained a crucial caveat to this prohibition that would form the basis of the legalization of *Ulysses* in 1933. It stated that 'the Secretary of the Treasury may, in his discretion, admit the so-called classics or books of recognized and established literary or scientific merit, but may, in his discretion, admit such classics or books only when imported for non-commercial purposes'.[17] The Tariff Act introduces the possibility of immunity from seizure and prosecution any text that comes under the category of a 'classic' or one that can be considered of sufficient literary worth so as to exonerate its sexual content.[18] But these categories of 'classic' and 'literary merit' were not defined by the act itself, necessitating further precedent as to discern their legal meaning. It was this clause, however, that gave hope to the legal team tasked with defending Joyce's text because they believed that they could persuasively argue that *Ulysses* met these criteria and could thus be imported into the United States.

Before moving to the legal team's strategies and arguments, it is necessary to examine another aspect of American law that motivated both Joyce and his legal team to attempt to overturn the ban on *Ulysses*: American copyright law. Following the guilty verdict in *The Little Review* trial, Joyce found it impossible to find a publisher for *Ulysses* in both America and Britain, leading him eventually to have the text published in France with Sylvia Beach's Shakespeare and Company. Although small, Shakespeare and Company did not have a reputation for the distribution of pornography leading to the hope on Joyce and Beach's parts that a copyright for the text could be attained in the United States. However, the Chace Act 1891 that set down the terms for English language publication copyrights in America contained a crucial manufacturing clause that stipulated that in order to be eligible for copyright protection, a text must be produced in the States themselves by American printing presses. It was not the fact that *Ulysses* was deemed obscene that prevented Joyce from attaining copyright but rather that a mainstream publisher feared prosecution after publishing the text in America that prevented Joyce attaining copyright protection. Unable to secure protection for his text and with copies now available for Americans to purchase from France lead to a situation wherein, as Robert Spoo describes, 'the copyright code, the obscenity law, and customs officials [...] combined to strip Joyce of his literary property in America.[...] *Ulysses* had entered the public domain—prematurely, but nonetheless surely'.[19] Any publisher could thus publish an unexpurgated edition of *Ulysses* immune from financial responsibilities to Joyce and immune from prosecution in the courts.

The man to take up this opportunity was Samuel Roth, who, in many ways, takes up a similarly ambivalent position to both the sexual deviant publisher of high modernism and the figure of the gangster, both criminal and public servant. Roth has similarly been figured as both purveyor of low pornography and purloiner of author's income and at the same time champion of the *avant-garde* and transgressor of wrongful laws. A writer and poet in his early life, Roth used funds gathered from his school for teaching English to immigrants to fund a number of literary magazines, which could, in his own words, 'give artistic expression to the ideas and emotions of my time'.[20] One of those magazines was *Two World's Monthly* in which Roth decided to publish the 1922 edition of *Ulysses* without the consent of Joyce or any financial dividends towards the author. The name itself, as Spoo describes, signifies both a commitment to the transgressions of national boundaries as well as 'the provocative heterogeneity of Roth's magazine, with its nervous oscillation between literary ambition and bawdy entertainment'.[21] The first edition appeared in 1925 and was dedicated to Joyce and contained pirated editions of both Ezra Pound and an early part of Joyce's *Work in Progress* lifted from *The Criterion*, all of which had no copyright protection in the United States due to the manufacturing clause of the Chace Act.

Roth began issuing unauthorized instalments of *Ulysses* in *Two Worlds* in July 1926. In response, Joyce and Beach organized at first Ezra Pound's idea of a "firmly abusive campaign in the press", in which Roth and his publication were firmly denounced in every publication that would let them publish. The aim was to attack Roth's credibility in New York in the hope that this pressure would force him to stop printing *Ulysses* as well as build Joyce's reputation as an author of literary merit who, once again, was the victim of injustice. When this failed to stop Roth, Beach organized an international protest in 1927 in which a litany of contemporary authors signed a letter in support of Joyce and denouncing Roth's piracy as well as the laws that facilitated this perceived injustice.[22] This again was followed by an attempt at injunction against Roth for the misappropriation of Joyce's name which was successful. The entire Roth episode would come to play a key part in the coming trial of 1933 and had set about changing the public perception of both Joyce and his text. As Spoo states:

> By presenting himself as a sufferer under American law, Joyce rewrote a narrative that had cast him as the law's subverter; [...]In the wake of Joyce's revisionary campaign, *Ulysses* came to seem more sinned against than sinning, less a corrupter of morals than a scene of trespass. Fashioning himself as an aggrieved rights holder and his book as a vandalized temple, Joyce laid the groundwork for the eventual authorized edition of *Ulysses* in the United States.[23]

It is also apparent how the figure of Joyce, the author of the text, comes to be the means by which the text's transition from obscenity to legitimacy takes place. We have a case of *Ulysses* the legitimate work of art and its pirated double upon whom the suspicion that once came over the former is displaced onto the latter: Roth takes the place of the obscene pornographer that the name of Joyce once occupied. The support garnered by Beach's protest, as well as the international recognition of *Ulysses* as a work of high literary merit, would be considered as evidence for the legal team in the coming trial. This recognition, they would argue, was evidence that *Ulysses* was both a work of significant literary merit and held the status of a classic, both of the provisos necessary for a text to be allowed entry into the nation under the 1930 Tariff Act. The injunction against Roth and the public attention garnered by the protest also opened up a new market for a publisher to capitalize on Joyce's text.

In 1931, both Random House and Viking Press, who had just secured the rights for publishing what would become *Finnegans Wake*, began to explore the potential avenues for publishing an American edition of *Ulysses*. Both publishers, while in negotiations with Joyce, secured the services of the legal firm of Greenbaum, Wolff & Ernst who in the past decade had built a reputation for combatting obscenity accusations with mostly positive results. The firm themselves were keen to take the case on, with Alex Lindey, an attorney at the firm, stating in an office memorandum that he felt 'very keenly that this would be the grandest obscenity case in the history of law and literature'.[24] The text and the name of Joyce were both valued very highly by the firm, a value they believed would transfer onto them if the book was cleared, but they also felt that the text would be valuable for America itself.

The firm first had to contend with the proviso that a text could not be granted immunity if it was allowed in for commercial reasons. In a letter to Ben Huebsch of Viking Press, Morris Ernst, who would take control of the text's defence, advised that this would not be an issue due to Roth's previous pirating of the novel: 'From a monetary point of view, it is now a valueless commodity in the United States except for a few isolated pirates'.[25] As we have seen, the category of pornography and the form of enjoyment it is presupposed to elicit is continually attached to its status as a commodity and its availability on the market. By removing the potential monetary value of *Ulysses*, the defence could focus on the ways in which the text, as a work of literature, could elicit a different form of enjoyment from the reader.

The problem of the commercial intent of the publishers could also be elided by having a single text, ostensibly for private use, seized by customs and subsequently challenged in the courts. If this challenge was successful, then the text would no longer be deemed obscene under the Tariff Act, and further issues could then be issued from Paris. As for the subsequent publishing of the book in America, there were fears on the part of publishers that even if *Ulysses* were to receive a favourable ruling in New York, this ruling would not be binding for any other State and would lead to a number of further trials in each respective State, which would be a costly and potentially felonious enterprise for any potential publisher.[26] The firm's response to this issue was to recommend to the publisher that any positive legal decision should be printed as a foreword to any forthcoming publication:

> The method we have usually employed to retard independent State action is to write a foreword in the American edition, setting forth [...] the favourable opinion of the Court.
>
> You will note that in the American editions of *Married Love*, [...] *The Well of Loneliness* [and *The*] *Decameron*, forewords which we have prepared so that the volume itself, if ever hailed into court again would contain within its own pages, legal opinions and literary comment otherwise inadmissible in a court trial.[27]

By adding the favourable legal decision as a foreword, the legal trial would have to consider that decision as part of the text as a whole, making it very difficult to convincingly argue that a text was obscene when that text contained evidence that it was definitively not.

But more than this practical use of the foreword to stave off prosecution, this strategy is also indicative of a larger tactic of transforming the meaning of the text itself and re-figuring and ultimately policing the form of enjoyment garnered from the text itself. After victory in the trial, Ernst would write that the legal argument had allowed the text to finally 'speak for itself'.[28] But, in order for the text to be able to speak its truth, significant editing of the textual body and supplementary critical material was required to do so. And in doing this, the potentially dangerous, intoxicating aspect of the text could be elided. Thus, to speak its inner truth, the body of the text requires the insertion of that which is outside it. Avital Ronelll notes a similar dynamic in the writing of the experience of drugs wherein in order to describe the essence of the experience, a citation is required:

> Drugs [...] are animated by an outside already inside. [...] Benjamin takes an injection of a foreign body (Baudelaire's *Les Paradis artificiels*) in order to express his inner experience. This is by no means an atypical gesture. Thomas De Quincey cited Wordsworth. These texts are on each other. A textual communication based on *tropium*.[29]

The truth which demands to be spoken, the truth of the subject or of the text, can only be done through the medium of the other. So that in amending the text of *Ulysses* in order to protect it from accusations of being a corrupting agent, in order that its truth be revealed, the act itself testifies to the text's impotence to do so and its potential to be read and enjoyed in other manners. As I have noted above, those illicit forms of enjoyment perceived in the literary text and intoxicating substances are linked to the problem of truth, those substances come to signify a form of pleasure taken in untruth; what is being injected in *Ulysses* is in another way an immunization of that pleasure, a dose of truth, the truth of the text verified by the university and legitimated by the law itself.[30] But again, the necessity of these statements of truth by critic and judge bring into question both the stable meaning of the text being argued for and, by extension, the ability of the law itself to adequately define the truth.

This strategy of textual supplementation and transformation would prove decisive for the legal team who, in preparation for the case, went to work both altering the text of *Ulysses* itself and collecting other texts for inclusion in their briefs and to send to the judge who would later read the novel. The initial plan to begin legal proceedings was to arrange for a copy of *Ulysses* to be sent from Paris to New York and to inform the customs department of its arrival to ensure it would be seized. But before sending the text, Ernst recommended that a number of critical readings of the text be pasted into the text in order that they too would be considered part of the text as a whole and provide some semblance of order to the original text. If it could be argued that the text was in fact ordered, this would allow the defence to posit that the text was designed with artistic intent and that the function of that order was to reproduce a form of order found in the world itself: in short, their argument would be that *Ulysses* was a true reproduction of modern life and, as such, had a relation to truth that would garner it the classification of a modern classic and absolve it of the suspicion of obscene untruth and the pleasure associated with that untruth.

After these textual alterations were in place, Ernst and Lindey set about gathering their own critical texts and data on *Ulysses*. Knowing that witnesses would not be allowed to give evidence, the legal team decided to send out 500 letters to 'eminent people' asking 'their opinions on *Ulysses*'.[31] These opinions would be cited in Ernst's brief which would be sent to the judge presiding over the case. The letter itself reveals the degree to which expertise in literary studies was to be mobilized by the defence:

> We realize that the success of the attempt will depend [...] upon the extent to which intelligent and qualified public opinion can be rallied to the

> defense of the book. [...] What we would like to have is not so much a strict literary appraisal, as an estimate of the novel as a social document.[32]

The defence thus attempts to garner the opinion of the public in order to demonstrate that the law itself does not reflect the will of the people. But in much the same way as letting the text speak for itself by having others speak for it, the will of the people must be spoken by those 'intelligent and qualified' enough to do so. Qualified, here, works in two ways, it presupposes an authority and knowledge of the text being discussed, an authority granted by the power relations inherent within both academia and the literary zones. By virtue of their positions, these people are thus qualified to speak the truth of *Ulysses* and have their truth valued more highly than that of someone reading outside of these institutions. But the very opinion desired from the defence is also qualified in the sense that they would prefer an evaluation of the text that is not literary but one that testifies to the text as a 'social document'. By figuring *Ulysses* as a social document, the text can thus be positioned as part of the polis, engaging with society and facilitating the reader's engagement with the polis also. The truth that is demanded of the text is thus already qualified so as to eliminate the 'literary' aspect, which introduces the problem of the use value of literature and the solitary enjoyment it elicits, in preference for a form of truth that emphasizes *Ulysses* as a reflection of society. Through this act of truthful reproduction, shorn of any literary excess, the text's immunity can be justified.

The responses were in keeping with the request. Poet and critic Louis Untermeyer wrote that:

> it seems incredible [...] that, in these days of organized lawlessness, there should be a law that operates against masterpieces of art. [...]What Freud is to modern psychology, or Einstein to our revised notions of time and space, *Ulysses* is to the novel.[33]

John Dos Passos responded by arguing that:

> Since it deals with human life it can't very well help having some smut in it. [...] As a picture of Dublin it's a picture of any modern city, as a picture of Bloom and Stephen it gives you the very essence of the internal struggle on the dying middle class; that one Dublin day is a microcosm of the lives of hundreds of millions of *hommes moyen sensuels* of Western civilization.[34]

And F. Scott Fitzgerald stated that '[c]ompared to the pornography on the newsstands *Ulysses* is an Elsie Book' and that the '[p]eople who have the patience to read *Ulysses* are not the kind who will slobber over a few Rabelaisian passages'.[35] These three responses all enter *Ulysses* into varying economies wherein the text gains its value via comparison to another object. *Ulysses* gains its worth for Untermeyer by its proximity to Einstein and Freud, names which signify here innovation and the discovery of truth. For Dos Passos, the text's value is again its proximity to truth: the faithful representation of life demands 'some smut', but the act of authentic representation redeems the sexual aspect by making it subservient to truth. Likewise, the text's depiction of Dublin, Bloom and Stephen allows for identification from any average man in Western civilization, thus marking the text out as a social document invested and imbricated in the polis.[36] Fitzgerald's defence of the book requires the introduction of an imagined piece of pornography against which *Ulysses*' value is gained not from it nearness but from its perceived distance. This distance is so great that *Ulysses* is posited as closer in kind to Martha Finley's Elsie Dinsmore series of books for children than to pornography. Once again, the figure of the child, an assumedly female child, is invoked as the sexless opposite to the pornographic text and a potential victim of that text's sexuality. But whereas before the Young-Girl was figured as a potential victim of *Ulysses*, here Joyce's text is identified with that role, figuring the text as both sexless and innocent: the strategy for the defence of a text is the positing of a scapegoat text upon which the stain of improper enjoyment can be transferred.

These three responses are instructive in that they represent the overall strategy for the defence of *Ulysses*: it is a classic, its status as a classic is recognized by experts, selected guardians of truth, and any potentially pornographic enjoyment to be gained by reading the text is defused by both the text's difficulty and its commitment to truth.

In order to better justify these experts' opinions, the defence also sent out a questionnaire to over 800 libraries asking if the libraries in question stocked a copy of *Ulysses*, how much demand there was for the text and if the librarian themselves supported the legal team's attempt to decriminalize the text. The responses were, again, mostly supportive of the defence's potential action and many declared that they were in possession of a copy of *Ulysses*. Those who were not supportive were therefore removed from the pool of data being accumulated, attesting to the careful manipulation of this data in order to make their expert opinions, and the public will match their argument. With this data, the defence could argue three interconnected points: first, if national and public libraries across America were in possession of the text, then this would evidence that the law was unsuccessful. Second, if copies of *Ulysses* were available in America, then this had not seen a concomitant detrimental effect on the readers of the text and the nation as a whole; therefore, the law was also unnecessary. Third, if there was a genuine demand for the text from the public for an item that had no provable harmful effects then not only was the law unsuccessful and unnecessary but it was also unjust.

As if to prove the first point, the copy of *Ulysses* sent from Paris was initially allowed through customs despite the tip off from Ernst. The copy had to be sent back and customs reminded of its status as contraband before it was eventually seized and this seizure was challenged. Ernst decided that it would be best to avoid a jury trial, ostensibly to avoid the time and costs that would be accrued waiting for each member of the jury to read the text.[37] The team were however willing to delay the case until they could guarantee 'a favourable and liberal judge' to read and decide upon the text.[38] This move is another example of the careful management of the case by Ernst and Lindey, aware that in order for *Ulysses* to speak for itself, they'd require a judge who was willing to listen to it and let them translate what it said: Woolsey, ultimately, was judged by them to be more open to influence, more likely to be seduced by a strategically presented critical consensus on the text's meaning.

Woolsey decided that if he were to pass judgement on the text, then he should carefully read the text over the summer of 1932. Whilst this was in process, the defence supplied Woolsey with both Stuart Gilbert's 1930 study of the text and Paul Jordan Smith's *A Key to Ulysses* in a further attempt to convince Woolsey of the consensus among experts of the literary value and underlying order within *Ulysses*. Both Gilbert and Smith's studies lean upon supplementary texts in order to validate their truth claims: Gilbert's study depends heavily upon the Gilbert Schema provided to him by Joyce in 1921, and this schema was also used by Ernst and Lindey in their arguments for the order of *Ulysses*. Smith's study leans upon a map of Dublin to trace the events of the text. In both cases, the literary text's truth depends upon a deferral to another text upon which a truth claim can be more comfortably grounded and in that process repressing the supplementary text's status as text, as susceptible to the ambiguity of the signifier as that which it seeks to clarify. A map would also be produced for the defence in which the libraries that stocked *Ulysses* were plotted in order to demonstrate the presence of the foreign body of the text within the national body: one of the key strategies for the defence was the accumulation of empirical data with which they could supplement the text, thus offsetting the non-being potential untruth within the text itself. But this act requires a form of disavowal, a specific fetish relation to data that renounces the data's existence as a signifier in the name of a form of enjoyment, an enjoyment in truth. The enjoyment of data as truth is thus founded upon the very same basis as the enjoyment in non-truth, fantasy. The defence are thus figuring the text not as a medium for fantasies of untruth but as a catalyst for a shared enjoyment of truth and an essential correlation between signifier, signified and referent: what I have elsewhere referred to as the fantasy of the sexual relation. Contrary to the previous trials, the literary text is being here figured as an ally to the sexual relation, and, crucially, the law's intervention will be figured as harmful to life itself.

This is the strategy of Ernst's brief delivered to the court: it is the law that needs to change to accommodate *Ulysses* and the form of life it represents, the life of the average man in 1932. His brief is, like their modified copy of *Ulysses*, a hybrid text composed of legal argumentation and citations of precedent and literary criticism, detailing the importance and value of Joyce's novel. Here, we have an instance wherein literary criticism and legal discourse no longer conflict but form an alliance to offer a mutual claim to truth. But in order to do so, Ernst had to figure *Ulysses*, Joyce, and the past censorship of the text in a particular fashion so as to both convince Woolsey of the truth of his argument and as to the injustice Joyce had suffered under the previous law.

His first line of argument was that *Ulysses* constituted an exceptional and, critically, modern text that demanded to be judged carefully by the existing law, and, if necessary, the law would need to change to accommodate it. Ernst begins his brief by stating

> [c]ourts have often been called upon to pass upon books, but never upon a work of the magnitude and newness, of the complexity, of the literary importance of *Ulysses*. The book is unlike any other work that has preceded it. [...] There is every reason, therefore, why the rules of law which are invoked in ordinary cases, should be applied here with exceptional circumspection.[39]

Ulysses is thus figured not in terms of sexuality but rather in terms of complexity, modernity and as an event in literary production that renders the text unique. Its status as a unique exception in literature demands an exceptional status within legal discourse also. *Ulysses* both requires expertise from both its readers and its legal assessors.

After arguing for the text's exceptional character, Ernst then goes on to describe the character of Joyce and his exceptional place in literary history. He begins his character analysis by distinguishing Joyce from other Irish writers:

> Unlike Shaw and others of his countrymen Joyce has steadfastly scorned ballyhoo and self-exploitation. He has led a monastic existence [...]. Nearly as blind as the Greek master from whose epic he borrowed the name of his novel, he has lived apart, an austere Olympian.

Joyce is thus presented in comparison to other Irish writers in much the same manner as *Ulysses* to pornography. Other Irish writers have sullied themselves with manipulation of the public for money, whereas Joyce has only wanted to produce art and is thus ridden of the corruption associated with the market. His 'austere' and 'monastic' life figures him in terms of sobriety and control, again disassociating him from the destructive excess enjoyment associated with intoxicating substances.[40] Joyce himself is also presented as a father to a new method of literary production, with Ernst arguing that 'there is not a single psychological novel worthy of mention that does not bear some trace of the Joycean method'.[41] Joyce's value as an author can thus be measured in modern literature's debt to him to accuse *Ulysses* of obscenity is thus to accuse all modern literature of the same crime. This is also evidence of the use value of the text, it has had an effect on other subjects and has been used by them, thus functioning as evidence for the text as a social document rather than a strictly literary one, absolving the texts of all the suspicions that the law previously attached to the latter.

The comparison to Homer, however, signals a different co-extensive, if contradictory, strategy. As well as framing *Ulysses* as an exception, Ernst also attempted to contextualize Joyce as the latest, and greatest, writer in a long tradition of western literature. Mobilizing a litany of citations from literary critics the brief detail's favourable comparisons to Dante, Flaubert, Balzac, Zola, Swift, Goethe, Dostoevsky and Henry James. By co-opting Joyce in with these names, the author and by extension his text gain their value from their proximity to these names and the distance in time: his place in a tradition comes to signify not a solitary and masturbatory form of writing but a link with a fantasy of an unbroken cultural heritage from Ancient Greece to 1930s America. Placing the text in this tradition, within a fantasmatic structure of contiguous white, male identity, allows for Joyce to play the part of the sole living representative of that tradition. If Woolsey and other legal professionals were invested in that fantasy, then to attack Joyce was to disrupt and discredit this collective white male identity. This implicit gendering of the text is important because, by figuring the text as the product of a male tradition and presenting Joyce as a father, the enjoyment of the text is no longer associated with female readers and their associated feminine *jouissance*: by putting *Ulysses* in a masculine context, the enjoyment of the text is figured as phallic enjoyment rather than the feminine, queer or Other enjoyment that the text had previously been associated with.

But a tension emerges here: Ernst's claims to the source of the text's value contradict: on the one hand, *Ulysses*' value and importance derive from its modernity, as an exception from past novels; on the other hand, the text's value can be proved by its presence within a long tradition of literary production which has been recognized as valuable to the ongoing progress of civilization. This tension is not resolved in Ernst's brief, and it is interesting the degree to which the literary text is allowed to exist within this undecidable space where its value and truth is grounded on shifting and contradictory sources, whereas, as I will discuss below, the law itself must meet the demands of modernity. This double and thus impossible source of value attests to a dimension of the literary text which the attempt to name its truth is designed to deny. And it is the discourse of literary criticism that, in Ronell's formulation, functions as the article that covers the literary text's work and provides the grounds upon which the law can do its own work.[42] It is upon the claims of criticism that Joyce's reputation is produced and upon this reputation that Ernst can claim that 'It is monstrous to suppose that a man of the stature of Joyce would or could produce a work of obscenity'.[43] And in doing so frames the trial in terms of morality, whereby the law, and not the text, is accused of monstrosity. Because, despite the contradictions, both of the grounds upon which Joyce's value is posited place his name and his text firmly on the side of life, with all the moral associations that come with that concept. By figuring *Ulysses* as the quintessentially modern text, this modernity comes to signify the text's fidelity to modern life, that which exists at this very moment. And by framing Joyce as the descendant of a long literary tradition, another aspect of life can be mobilized: reproduction.[44] Both Joyce's relation to modernity and his place in a tradition come to signify the text's relation to vitality. The figure of the author, framed either way, is a necessary supplement in order to fix the text's truth and remove its potentially intoxicating effects.

This manoeuvre allows Ernst to cast the law in the opposite role, as anti-life. He does this initially by contrasting the modernity of the world *Ulysses* is purported to represent and exist within against the anachronism of obscenity law. He first begins by disputing the use of 19th-century standards to judge literary texts in the 1930s. He states that 'what is decent or indecent is determined by the sensibilities and moral standards of the people, as evolved from generation to generation along with their civilization'.[45] In the same way, the novel has evolved with civilization and found its zenith in *Ulysses*, so must the law continue to evolve lest it commit an injustice not only against the text but also to civilization. Ernst continues to emphasize the need for a law attuned to the contemporary moment and not the past by quoting previous precedent set by Judge Learned Hand wherein he argues for a more modern and flexible standard for obscenity: 'should not the word "obscene" be allowed to indicate the *present critical point* in the compromise between candour and shame at which the community may have arrived *here and now*?'.[46] In this sense, the category of obscenity is not fixed but constantly shifting necessitating a law attuned to these shifts and willing to reproduce the will of the community in its judgements. And again, the emphasis here is on the present, upon modernity as the source of value for not only literature but also the law.

As to these contemporary standards of morality, Ernst argues that 'the standards of yesterday, the abhorrence of any mention of certain biological functions, the excessive prudery, the sex taboo, are as definitely dead today as the horse-drawn carriage and the donkey engine'.[47] Contemporary America is thus presented as an enlightened culture unafraid of sexuality and eager to confront it. The past, and its associated investments in secrecy, is framed as 'excessive' and 'dead', with the contemporary moment presented as the bearer of life and truth. The past cultural mores are compared to now obsolete technologies and are similar in both their deadness, their lack of utility and their replacement by more modern forms. The effect of this comparison is the production of an historical impetus that is compelling the perpetual growth and evolution of civilization. The challenge to the law thus set by *Ulysses* as modernist text is also the challenge set by America of the 1930s. Ernst's challenge to the law is the modernist challenge to art: make it new. Ernst is asking for a form of law determined by the present and not the past. But, whereas in the case of *Ulysses* and the literary tradition, the past is a source of value and evidence of the text's vitality; here, the past is the realm of the dead and obsolete. But within Ernst's discourse that emphasizes the contemporary commitment to truth, that very commitment to confronting sexuality is itself undercut by Ernst's use of language, denigrating the past's prudery whilst refusing to name the 'biological functions' he claims are now discussed openly. Operative within Ernst's discourse of truth is the same form of veiling that his discourse is claiming to combat.

Ernst's evidence for contemporary America's lack of shame and commitment to truthful representation is the press. Contrasting the practices of the past with contemporary journalism, Ernst states that:

> Our tabloids carry stories of passion and lust, of crime and perversion, told with a degree of graphic vividness unheard of a generation ago. Every man, woman and child in the community has easy access to the complete details of torch-murders, marital infidelities, of boudoir intimacies, of kidnappings and abnormalities. [...] For the press today a spade is a spade. No longer are such squeamish phrases as "statutory offence" resorted to. The headlines and the columns speak openly of rape, blood-lust and adultery.[48]

The newspapers of contemporary America are depicted as texts in which practices which are perceived to embody destructive forms of enjoyment are represented freely. These texts are themselves available to women and children, the readership who have previously been understood as most at risk from the dissemination of pornographic texts. But what redeems these texts, what makes them contemporary and gives them their value, is their commitment to the truth, to call 'a spade a spade', and to represent the world with the correct signifiers and not to use 'squeamish phrases' where other more accurate descriptions will do. What defines the contemporary era is fidelity to the truth and the true representation of life itself. Even potentially harmful practices and substances can be mitigated if their uses and representations can be justified according to this duty thus ridding them of the suspicion of improper enjoyment in untruth or destruction.

After depicting both *Ulysses* and the contemporary society that the novel was said to represent, Ernst then depicted the law that governed both. Ernst begins by returning to *R v Hicklin* and the test for obscenity that dominated all subsequent obscenity trials. The Hicklin test is referred to as 'the ancient test', immediately disassociating it from the modernity celebrated in the previous paragraphs.[49] The precedent set down in Hicklin that set forth that the criterion for obscenity was a text's perceived effect on a vulnerable reader was both unjust and obsolete by the standards of 1930s America:

> Such a criterion was patently unfair, unreasonable, and unsound, because it sought to gauge the moral and mental capacity of the community by that of its dullest witted and most fallible members, and because it sought to withhold from society any material which might conceivably injure its lowest and most impressionable element.[50]

By setting the imagined figure of the most vulnerable and impressionable as the test for obscenity, Ernst argues that the Hicklin test unjustly punishes those that are not vulnerable to corruption. The Hicklin test encourages the creation of fantasy figures such as the Young-Girl in *The Little Review* trial, which quickly become a screen for multiple libidinal investments and prevented the law from appreciating the text and its effect on the aggregate population, on whose part the law is supposed here to work. *Hicklin*, according to this argument, may appear to help those most vulnerable, but, in doing so, damages civilization by preventing it access to materials that could be used for its own improvement. The law, by focusing on the lowest common denominator, is thus damaging the progress of civilization as a whole and thus to modern life. By framing the law as anti-life, the *pharmakon* of the text can thus appear as a source of life. The *pharmakon* in this context becomes the means by which the polis can be rejuvenated. This positive aspect of the *pharmakon* is maintained by positioning the *pharmakon* as a victim of injustice, of misuse by a minority and misunderstanding by the law. What is required of the law, and of Woolsey himself, is an 'enlightened definition of obscenity'. The use of enlightenment by Ernst implicitly historicizes Hicklin into an obsolete and ignorant period, as dead as the mores it represented, thus figuring the contemporary law that holds to that precedent as in need of the light and knowledge that *Ulysses* contains.[51]

This enlightened form of law must, Ernst argues, coincide with the will and mores of the people it seeks to represent: it must be on the side of life. With reference to the depictions of life in both the press and the arts, Ernst posits a new criterion for obscenity: 'Considering all the other influence and stimuli of modern life, the press, the stage, the movies, could the book really hurt a *normal* human being? For it is the *normal* person who must serve as a criterion'.[52] The average person in 1930s America, due to the time's commitment to truth, is thus more enlightened and by extension responsible than is considered in the Hicklin test. But for all its rhetorical force, Ernst's positing of a new criterion is in itself replacing one fantasy figure, the vulnerable Young-Girl, with another, the responsible and well-informed man. And as we have seen, the recourse to normality is itself bolstered by empirical data presented to the court, but this data has itself been managed in order to produce a certain truth: the norm that the data is supposed to support pre-exists the collation and management of that data. Still at work here is fantasy, however, instead of a fantasy that conceives of the *pharmakon* as a threat to social stability, here, the *pharmakon* is a source of power and vitality, it can be put to use in the name of the fantasy rather than against it. Crucial here however is the maintenance of the average man as a norm against which abnormality can be measured: excess must still be supressed, but it becomes now the responsibility of the subject and not the law to do so.

The excess that needs to be repressed is still evident in the defence's handling of the sexuality of the text. Sex can be tolerated if put to some use either for civilization or in the name of the continuation of life. But in order to put sex to work in the name of truth, this sexuality must be relegated to a function, a fact of life that the text must faithfully represent out of duty rather than enjoyment. Ernst's characterization of *Ulysses* and the presence of sexuality within it firmly demote sexuality under the authority of truth and life: according to Ernst, *Ulysses* is 'a many faceted crystallization of life and thought [...] Sex is present, to be sure, but sex is part of man's existence. One can no more say that *Ulysses* is obscene than that life or thought is obscene'.[53] Only as an aspect of the average man's life is sex allowed a place within the text. It is not the presence of sexuality that is presented as in itself obscene, but it becomes a question of quantity and intensity, measuring a normative relation to sexuality in order to gauge the normality of the subject's enjoyment of the text. Life and thought are thus posited as sets in which sexuality is contained, and the presence of sexuality in these sets does not threaten to corrupt and usurp these categories and transform them into obscenity as long as these sets are faithfully represented. The absence of corruption is predicated upon these categories being fixed and the relation to sexuality remaining normative. An excess of sexuality threatens the very vitality that its representation guarantees. Thus, a range of supplements such as truth and authorial intention are required in order to intervene in order to successfully maintain sex's place within the domain of life, but at the same time, this requirement for intervention indicates the trace of the destructive aspect of sex identified in previous trials as well as the Hicklin test against which the normal reader is now posited. Sex is still a threat to the average man as it was to the Young-Girl; the use of a norm, however, affords more means to manage, measure and put sex to work in a way that the prohibition did not. The *pharmakon*, properly managed, can thus be put to work in the name of the polis.

One way in which the *pharmakon* of *Ulysses* was mitigated was to categorize it as a classic thus conferring immunity for the text whilst also immunizing the text itself of its sexuality. Using the *Webster's Dictionary* definition of classic, Ernst states that '[t]he words "classic" and "obscenity" represent polar extremes. They are mutually antagonistic and exclusive. That which is obscene corrupts and depraves – it cannot be of the highest class and of acknowledged excellence'. Once again, a supplementary text is introduced in order to fix the truth of the literary text; this time, a text whose function is to stabilize the meaning of all signifiers and thus facilitate intersubjective communication. But even the dictionary definition is absent of the moral associations imparted by Ernst in his use of that definition: the definition introduces a special metaphor, but it is Ernst who interprets the definition of highest in terms of public good. What we witness here is not the declaration of an essential binary, but the production of an opposition by Ernst in order to qualify *Ulysses* on the side of the positive term: the supplementary text that is supposed to present objective knowledge is used in order to produce the effect of truth. A moral reading of the special metaphor must also be added to the definition in order for the binary between classic and obscenity to function. Ernst constantly introduces supplementary texts and assumptions in order to produce the desired truth effect of *Ulysses* whilst also presenting that truth as evidence. He argues that, in this trial, 'the sole evidence is the book', but at every step of the way, he is introducing supplementary evidence, texts and assumptions to prove the text's supposedly self-evident truth.

The figure of the average reader is mobilized in Ernst's brief in order to disqualify him from accessing the meaning of the text. Ernst argues that '[i]t is axiomatic that only what is understandable can corrupt', and he produces another binary opposition. By arguing that the reader must understand completely in order to be corrupted the meaning of that text, Ernst removes all transferential dynamics from the reading process instead positing the text as containing a fixed meaning that must be identified and then possessed by the reader. But the true meaning of *Ulysses* is not available to the average reader, who finds himself drastically unqualified for the task that the text sets him. The value of a reading of *Ulysses* is garnered only by its proximity to a pre-existing truth, any aspects of the reader's subjectivity that find themselves imbricated in his reading of the text are marked out as incoherent excesses, thus disqualifying the reading. Reading the text is thus presented as a detached practice, and the truth of the text figured as pure and sacred, in need of protection: the critic in this sense becomes a guardian of the text's truth against the masses. The institutional power of the university is thus mobilized in order to limit the power of the *pharmakon*, introducing both a moral and a political aspect into the argument that the representatives of the university have hegemony over the text's meaning. Ernst goes on to posit the presence of *Ulysses* on university reading lists as proof of the text's importance: 'It would be absurd to assume that an obscene work would appear as assigned reading in our institutions of learning'.[54] But also assumed here is the moral responsibility of the institution of the university for policing texts in service to the polis. Here the university is seen to be performing the same police function as the vigilance networks before them, with the added benefit of no longer requiring legal intervention. The critic's function is thus understood as a police function: policing both the morality of texts and their overall meaning. Part of this process is the production of an average reader and the production of his knowledge or its limits, limits which the critic can raise himself above in order to name them. By positing himself above the average man, it is also possible to theorize that this allows access to the obscene enjoyment of the text not granted to the average reader: the critic is thus granted a privileged space in which to enjoy the obscenity of the text on the condition that it remains within that space.

Ulysses, Ernst argues, presents numerous 'polysyllabic barriers' and 'countless passages which [...] appear to make no sense whatever'.[55] The linguistic experimentation of the text, the manner in which it transgresses linguistic norms does not, in turn, mark the text itself as transgressive; instead, this transgressive aspect comes to signify the text's impotence and function as the limit of understanding for the average reader. Rather than being too full of meaning, an excess that threatens the truth claim of the critic, the text is figured, for the average reader at least, as absent of meaning. In Ernst's argumentation, the average reader is incapable of understanding the truth of the text because even those most qualified of readers struggle. This is a view also held by Bennet Cerf who in a letter to Ernst states that 'dumbbells in search of smut will certainly throw down the book in hopeless disgust after trying to wade through the first two chapters'.[56] The average reader is figured as incapable of completing a journey through the text because he has misidentified the truth of the text. In a similar manoeuvre, Ernst argues that the value of *Ulysses* can only be ascertained, and the text can only be enjoyed once considerable work has been done both before and during the reading process:

> The book is treasure-trove, to be sure; but its riches are so well hid in grottoes of recondite learning, of classical allusions, of literary and scientific profundities, that the average seeker- blindly groping about in the surrounding maze- soon tires of the venture and turns back.[57]

The metaphor of a treasure chest that confers wealth upon a specialized cast of informed readers and leaves the 'average seeker' who lacks this knowledge incapable of profiting reproduces the economic and class relations operative in the university's production of knowledge: knowledge is produced within the university and access to it is regulated in order to maintain the class relations that allow for the conditions of its continuation. By virtue of being outside the university, the average reader is blind to the truth of *Ulysses*, which in turn figures the text as a means by which that exclusion can continue. Literary value takes on a very different meaning here, it is a means by which class relations are policed and maintained; the ability to perceive literary value of the truth of a text is proportional to one's social class. Far from threatening class relations, *Ulysses* can thus be weaponized in order to maintain them.

With the novel positioned as a faithful reflection of modern life, bestowed with the title of classic by the institutional power of the university and the average reader positioned as incapable of understanding the text, Ernst ends his brief by returning to the law and the challenges that modernity and *Ulysses* present to it. Arguing once more that the law's definition of obscenity should match the public's morality, Ernst states that:

> That which society accepts is moral; that which it rejects is immoral. The law must recognise and give effect to this principle, or else it becomes not a true mirror of life as it should be, but a bewildering distortion, alike perplexing and misleading, of which the ordinary man or woman becomes profoundly distrustful.[58]

The law must maintain its duty to represent in its own practice the morality of 'the ordinary man or woman'. Implicitly, the law, in regard to obscenity law, and the prior judgement of *Ulysses* in particular, has failed its duty. The metaphor of the mirror links this duty to represent to the perceived function of literature to reproduce truth, a form of truth that finds its veracity in the will of the people. Law that does not fulfil this mimetic function is perceived as untrue, perplexing and a distortion of the truth which is being figured here to pre-exist any legal decision. By arguing for this mimetic function, Ernst's reverses the accusations made by the law against the literary text. It is the law and not the text that embodies all the anxieties associated with untruth and the simulacrum. The law is here on the side of death, threatening social cohesion and collective identity. The literary text on the other hand, by virtue of its fidelity to truth, can be positioned on the side of life in that it facilitates this fantasy. In order to enact this reversal, Ernst has mobilized two supplements: the claim to truth and the average reader. The law is presented without supplements and, as such, occupy the position previously taken by the literary text as the dead letter, a form of writing divorced from the people it is supposed to represent, and the truth that they embody.

Woolsey took up this challenge whole-heartedly, and his decision is in itself an attempt to bring together the discourses of literary criticism and the law, just as Ernst had done in his brief. Woolsey's decision focused upon the text's relation to truth and the perceived intent behind the text and its imagined effect on a normal reader. But it is also a statement as to the truth of *Ulysses* and a declaration of his own reading prowess. He begins by stating that:

> *Ulysses* is not an easy book to read or to understand. But there has been much written about it, it is advisable to read a number of other books which have now become its satellites. The study of *Ulysses* is therefore a heavy task.[59]

Ulysses is thus conceptualized as a body around which critical works are massed, and to understand this body, these satellites must also be understood, and more than that, these subservient texts are in fact the sources of the meaning of the body around which they circulate. In this sense, Woolsey manages to elide the incoherence of *Ulysses*, an incoherence that once brought the text into disrepute, by giving legal recognition to the need for supplements in order to understand the novel. And in doing so legitimates the critic as the arbiter of the text's meaning and the university as the institution in which the text belongs. Woolsey thus begins his decision by agreeing with Ernst's implicit formulation of the critic's role in the production and policing of the truth.

Woolsey also introduces, justified by the introduction of literary merit as a condition of entrance in the Tariff Act, the previously inadmissible category of authorial intention. For Woolsey, if a book is to be found obscene, 'it must first be determined whether the intent with which it was written was [...] pornographic-that is, written for the purpose of exploiting obscenity'.[60] Therefore, obscenity can be present in the work but to what end that obscenity is put to work will determine whether a text is obscene. The pornographic text therefore is that which exploits obscenity for an intended effect that bears no relation to the truth: thus, Woolsey is in agreement with Ernst in that the presence of sex within a text is mitigated by virtue of the text's proximity to truth. This mitigation of sexuality by virtue of the text's perceived duty to truth is also evident when Woolsey declares that '[i]n spite of its unusual frankness, I do not detect the leer of the sensualist. I hold, therefore, that it is not pornographic'.[61] As is evident in my reading of *Ulysses* in chapter two, the *Nausicaa* chapter of the novel presents us with the image of a leering sensualist gazing upon a young woman as he masturbates.

Despite this representation of what is specifically defined by Woolsey as pornographic, the assumption of the novel's truth being located in the author's intention and not the words on the page that allows for the repression of potentially pornographic chapter. It is then the 'unusual frankness' of Joyce that facilitates this elision; the belief in the text's representation of truth allows for repression of the text's meaning. We can begin to postulate that the truth to which the text is dutiful is, like the Young-Girl of the previous trial, a fantasy object, a fantasy object that *Ulysses* is here facilitating access to instead of threatening to destroy.

The production of authorial intention as a means of fixing the text's meaning and domesticating the sexuality of the novel then allows Woolsey space to produce his own understanding of the novel:

> In writing Ulysses, Joyce sought to make a serious experiment in a new [...] literary genre. [...] Joyce has attempted- it seems to me, with astonishing success- to show how the screen of consciousness with its ever-shifting kaleidoscopic impressions carries, as if it were on a plastic palimpsest, not only what is in the focus of each man's observation of the actual things about him, but also in a penumbral zone residua of past impressions [...] drawn up by association from the domain of the subconscious.[62]

Joyce is here figured as a scientist attempting to render into words the truth of human consciousness. The success of this experiment, the correlation between the words and the truth, bestows upon the author and his text literary merit. But this supposed correlation requires the intervention of supplemental optic metaphors: consciousness is both a kaleidoscope and a palimpsest. Only once these optical supplements are in place can one conceive of the successful representation of the truth. Woolsey's recourse to the discourse of psychoanalysis is telling here also because the 'subconscious' is also posited as a realm of the subject's truth that the text records with fidelity, and that fidelity excuses any potential obscenity that emerges in the representation of the subconscious. It is an understanding of psychoanalysis as psychology, as a discourse of truth upon which truth claims can be legitimated. This discourse also functions as a supplement in the law's attempt to write about the truth of the text, betraying an insufficiency in both the text to simply represent the truth and the law to discern it.

This dependency on the insertion of supplementary discourses and media continues when Woolsey compares the novel to experimental film:

> What he seeks to get is not unlike the result of a double or, if that is possible, a multiple exposure on a cinema film which would give a clear foreground with a background visible but somewhat blurred and out of focus in varying degrees.[63]

Cinema is thus introduced in order to give stability to the text's meaning: the text is explained in terms of a film that bears the trace of multiple images occupying the same space, accounting in this comparison for the presence of multiple perspectives and discourses in the text. The film may appear 'blurred' and 'out of focus', but this instability is explained by the presence of multiple instances of the truth being recorded and the inability for the medium to reveal multiple images concurrently. Likewise, the multiple and competing discourses of the novel are only so many discourses of truth that find difficulty in being voiced at the same time and in the same language. But this, in a sense, admits to the failure of the medium in its aim. However, this failure is mitigated by its perceived intention: to represent the truth. Woolsey is aware of the conceptual difficulty in his comparison but uses this apparent dissonance in order to better explain the truth of the text. He argues that to 'convey by words an effect which obviously lends itself more appropriately to a graphic technique, accounts, it seems to me, for much of the obscurity which meets a reader of *Ulysses*'.[64] The image is thus depicted as the better medium for representing the truth, but the comparison, despite detailing the failure of Joyce's attempt, allows Woolsey to explain the obscurity of the text by virtue of an exterior supplement rather than by engaging with the potential meaning of those difficult parts. It is then the authorial fidelity to truth and the introduction of another medium that facilitate an understanding of *Ulysses* that manages to domesticate the previously seditious difficulty. Woolsey finishes his comparison by stating that '[i]f Joyce did not attempt to be honest in developing the technique which he has adopted in *Ulysses* the result would be psychologically misleading and thus unfaithful to his chosen technique. Such an attitude would be artistically inexcusable'. Art, in whatever medium, and however difficult, gains its value by virtue of its creator's perceived honesty and faith to truth. But the necessary introduction of the figure of the author, numerous critical texts, comparisons to different media, all in order to prove the text's truth content betrays the amount of work required to produce that very truth which is supposedly so apparent on the page. This work itself betrays a need or desire for that truth being produced, what we might call the addiction to truth operative in the critical and legal approaches to literary texts. The *pharmakon* may be being stripped of its seditious potential but is still no less addictive.

Such is the pharmacological function of Woolsey's decision: the introduction of this truth content to the *pharmakon* allows for a proportional reduction in the sexual aspect of the same object. In relation to the obscene words which constituted the majority of the prosecution's evidence against the book, Woolsey argued that Joyce's

> attempt sincerely and honestly to realize his objective has required him incidentally to use certain words which are generally considered dirty words and has led at times to what many think is a too poignant preoccupation with sex in the thoughts of his characters.[65]

Such incursions of sex in the text are misunderstood as excessive if the reader cannot detach their self from that particular instance and remain aware of the author's intention and the truth to which the text is intended to represent. With this knowledge, a knowledge produced not by the text, but outside and after it, these instances of sex become incidental, unfortunately necessary inclusions but nothing of major importance to the overall meaning of the text. Beginning his mobilization of the average reader, Woolsey adds that:

> The words which are criticized as dirty are old Saxon words known to almost all men and, I venture, to many women, and are such words as would be naturally and habitually used, I believe by the types of folk whose life, physical and mental, Joyce is seeking to describe. In respect of the recurrent emergence of the theme of sex in the minds of his characters, it must always be remembered that his locale was Celtic and his season Spring.[66]

Again, the fidelity to truth excuses any possible excessive investment in 'the theme of sex'. This is the case despite his character's displaying this very trait. In order to disqualify this stain of obscenity from the text, Woolsey mobilizes racial and zoological discourses by arguing that this excessive investment in sexuality is a trait of the Irish people themselves and intimates their nature as animalistic by referring to the mating season: by emphasizing spring as the season for the novel, Woolsey thus allows for the presence of sexuality to be both normalized and localized to a certain time and place as well as emphasizing the reproductive utility of the act itself. Sex has a time and a place in nature as it does in the novel. In order to complete this comparison, however, Woolsey once again has to misread the novel itself, reading the novel as set in the spring rather than the summer month of June. Such strategic misreading, and the introduction of exterior discourses, allows for the domestication of the text's sexuality. Woolsey finishes his discussion of the obscene words in the text by recourse to another visual medium:

> although it contains, as I have mentioned above, many words usually considered dirty, I have not found anything that I consider to be dirt for dirt's sake. Each word of the book contributes like a bit of mosaic to the detail of the picture which Joyce is seeking to construct for his readers.[67]

By conceiving of the text as a mosaic and every instance of sex as part of a larger picture, Woolsey emphasizes a form of reading that always maintains a perspective of a larger truth to which the fragmentary sex of the novel is being put to use. This mode of reading thus allows sex to be put to work in the name of this composite meaning, and by extension, the text can be put to work in the name of truth. Sexuality that does not work towards truth is thus presented as 'dirt for dirt's sake', and in framing it this way, one can perceive the disruptive potential of sex remains in Woolsey's analysis and, much like in the case of the production of truth content, the amount of work required by him and the prospective reader of *Ulysses* to delimit the sexual nature of the text. Sex and truth thus become opposed; one's ascendency marks the other's subservience to that cause: sex is either put to work for truth, or truth is destroyed by sex.

Commenting on Woolsey's decision, Wolfgang Streit argues that '[t]he central function of these verdicts is to establish the sexuality of *Ulysses* in the discursive sphere and to allow it to expand'.[68] The presence of sex within the novel is thus put to work in the name of truth by Woolsey and made into an area of enquiry for future readers. Woolsey shows himself capable of this sober detachment but he himself cannot be the criterion against which the obscenity of the text is judged. Therefore, a normative reader is introduced: 'Whether a particular book would tend to excite such impulses and thoughts must be tested by the Court's opinion as to its effect on a person with average sex instincts — what the French would call *l'homme moyen sensuel*'.[69] This average reader is not then measured by his intelligence but rather by the normality of his sexuality in both object and intensity. This signifies both an investment in maintaining a normative relation to sexuality, putting it to work but not investing excessively in it, and also a desire to police potential readers of *Ulysses*. As Streit states:

> under the guise of being a juridical statement on obscenity, the verdict purports to represent the normative authority on normality. It thus implicitly invites readers to scrutinize their reactions to the sexuality in the text. These reactions then become an indicator of the readers' own normality, thus exponentially expanding the territory of the will to knowledge.[70]

Any future reader, in order to discern their own relation to the norm, must conform to this manner of reading and reproduce it in order to access their own sexuality and demonstrate their normality. A desire is thus produced by the norm, the desire to conform to it which in turn creates a desire to read *Ulysses* in a manner which confirms that normality. This desire is founded upon a renunciation of sex in the name of truth to speak the truth of sex rather than sexualize the truth. The introduction of a norm manages to both introduce a new criterion for legal proceedings but also for reading *Ulysses*, with the text functioning as a test for sexual abnormality in its reader: the text is on the side of life insofar as it on the side of biopolitics, the management and codification of the life it is made to represent.

In creating this figure, Woolsey was aware of the potential criticism he would face if he declared himself a representative of normality when he states that 'the risk involved in the use of such a reagent arises from the inherent tendency of the trier of facts, however fair he may intend to be, to make his reagent too much subservient to his own idiosyncrasies'.[71] His answer to this problem was to give a copy of *Ulysses* to two of his personal friends who he does not name and ask them their opinions on the text. The only details Woolsey gives about these men is that '[t]hey are men whose opinion on literature and on life I value most highly'.[72] Their dual commitments to literature and life signal an understanding that these two categories are necessarily connected and that the value of literature is its proximity to life with obscenity signifying a commitment to sexuality and death. This description also implies that these readers possess the erudition supposedly required to make an assessment of the text: in this sense, neither of the three men would constitute an average reader of *Ulysses* in 1933. But Woolsey's definition of the normative reader only included his 'sex instincts', and Woolsey had already decided that both he and his two friends possessed a measured enough sexuality in order to soberly assess the text without fear of seduction. The results were as such:

> I was interested to find that they both agreed with my opinion: that reading "*Ulysses*" in its entirety, as a book must be read on such a test as this, did not tend to excite sexual impulses or lustful thoughts but that its net effect on them was only that of a somewhat tragic and very powerful commentary on the inner lives of men and women.[73]

The norm being created then requires the splitting of the sovereign into multiple assessors who together come to make a decision upon the text, thereby creating the norm and absolving the decision of the potentially arbitrary whims of the sovereign decision. But the extent to which these literary assessors differ in any substantial way from Woolsey, all three white, American, upper-middle class males, limits the degree to which separation can be achieved. The shared reading of the text by all three men provides a strategy of reading the text that emphasizes the text's relation to a larger instead of the sexuality of the text, by virtue of being a norm, and a norm sanctioned by the law itself, produces itself a legal demand to read the text in such a manner. Any deviation from this reading practice immediately singles out the reader, rather than the text, as sexually abnormal. For all the rhetoric of frankness and the absence of shame in discussion of sexuality in 1930s America, the anxieties that attend it still remain, but, in this process, the emphasis on policing that sexuality has shifted from the text and onto the subject, whose reading now transforms into a potential symptom of his improper enjoyment. The norm retains the same arbitrary violence of the legal decision; it is only more successful in offsetting the responsibility for maintaining that decision onto the subject. The law creating violence remains in the hands of the sovereign, and the law preserving violence is now the responsibility of the reader.

Further evidence of the figure of the sovereign operative behind the apparently objective norm is the absence of any citations by either the critics Woolsey mentions or the other two assessors who allow Woolsey to construct his norm and disavow the presence of his own 'idiosyncrasies' in his ruling. Commenting on this absence, Streit contends that 'by excluding the statements, Woolsey ensured that his verdict *en passant* could be proved by his own normality and that of the assessors he selected'.[74] The norm is thus a product of the sovereign decision, finding its legitimacy not in empirical data's self-evident truth, but in the sovereign decision of the law and its investment in maintaining fantasmatic investments in truth and order.

Woolsey finishes his decision with a return to the rhetoric of drugs, whose enjoyment can now be tempered and put to work in the name of truth. He states that:

> I am quite aware that owing to some of its scenes "*Ulysses*" is a rather strong draught to ask some sensitive, though normal, persons to take. But my considered opinion, after long reflection, is that whilst in many places the effect of "*Ulysses*" on the reader undoubtedly is somewhat emetic, nowhere does it tend to be an aphrodisiac.

"*Ulysses*" may, therefore, be admitted into the United States.[75]

Ulysses is compared to an alcoholic 'draught' of particular intensity for the average subject, potentially intoxicating. But with the requisite reading practices in place, a reading practice predicated on a dependency upon authorial intention, literary criticism and a pre-conceived truth that the text sincerely attempts to reproduce, the effects of the *pharmakon* be mitigated. In fact, the mitigation of these effects becomes itself desirable by the injunction to conform to the norm and confess any aberration thus rendering the *pharmakon* of use to the law and biopower rather than disrupting its effects. With these safeguards successfully produced and legitimized by the law, the *pharmakon*'s effect on the subject shift from the aphrodisiac effects previously in the previous trial is now diagnosed as an emetic effect. The aphrodisiac, inducing as it were an excessive investment in sex, would seem to collapse the differentiation between subject and other, inside and outside that is necessary for producing the truth of the text in this trial: the disruptive quality of sex is therefore figured as that which has to be contained by the law and the subject. An emetic function, conversely, maintains the distinction between the interior body and the foreign element being expelled into the exterior where it is designated to belong.

Instead of categorizing the essence of the text as emetic, however, it is also possible to describe the mode of reading favoured by both Ernst and Woolsey as emetic in fashion. The strategy of inserting exterior texts into the body of *Ulysses* in order to dispel the sexuality of the text is what allows for the meaning of the text to be fixed. By then, transferring this emetic process onto the text itself, as its truth, the work required to produce that truth is hidden. The truth of the text then comes to veil the process by which that truth is made, namely the dependence upon the supplements in order to let the text speak for itself.

Woolsey's decision would later be published as the foreword to the American edition of *Ulysses*, completing a process of insertion that had allowed for the truth of the text to be fixed, thus allowing the law to deem the text no longer obscene. But also the decision itself, as the initial text a new reader of *Ulysses* would encounter would not only deter future obscenity litigation against the text but also introduce the reader to an understanding of the sexuality of the text in a detached and discursive manner, inciting in the reader to adhere to the normative reading of the text and police their own enjoyment of the novel.

Notes

1 U.S. Constitution Amend. XXI, Sec. 2.
2 John M. Woolsey, quoted in *The United States Vs One Book Called Ulysses by James Joyce: Documents and Commentary – A Fifty Year Perspective*, (Frederick, MD: University Publications of America, 1984), p. 38.
3 Avital Ronell, *Crack Wars: Literature Adiction, Mania*, (London: University of Illinois Press, 2004), p. 57.
4 The *pharmakon* of alcohol, just as the *pharmakon* of the obscene text, is posited as a potential danger to ~~The~~ Woman, the fantasy upon which so much is libidinally invested. At this particular moment, in American history, alcohol poses a threat to the sexual relation, or perhaps, stands as evidence of the non-existence of that relation.
5 Anne Wittenmyer, The *History of the Woman's Temperance Crusade*, (Boston, MA: James Earle, 1882), p. 21.
6 Ibid. p. 28.
7 Georges Bataille, *The Accursed Share, An Essay on General Economy, Volume One: Consumption*, (New York: Zone Books, 1991), p. 119.
8 Michael Lerner, *Dry Manhattan: Prohibition in New York City*, (London: Harvard University Press, 2011), p. 30.
9 Antonio Gramsci, 'America and Fordism', in *The Gramsci Reader: Selected Writings 1916–1935*, (New York: New York University Press, 2000), pp. 275–300, p. 280. In this essay, Gramsci argues that this transformation of the subject's relation to work and sexuality is a necessary precondition for a future transition to communism also.
10 Ibid. p. 286.
11 Daniel Bell, *The Cultural Contradictions of Capitalism*, (New York: Basic Books, 1996), p. 64.
12 Rachel Potter, *Obscene Modernism: Literary Censorship and Experiment 1900–1940*, (Oxford: Oxford University Press, 2013), p. 21.
13 Dirk Van Hulle, *James Joyce's 'Work in Progress': Pre-book Publications of Finnegans Wake Fragments*, (London: Routledge, 2016), p. 184.
14 The lack of funding for policing of alcohol and obscene texts was a constant point of contention during this period signalling an official commitment to protecting Americans from these evil substances, but a significant lack of political will to follow through on these commitments.
15 Tariff Act of 1930: § 1305. Accessed 31/07/18.
16 The specific laws for alcohol, which would act as a fourth source of illicit enjoyment, are found in a separate portion of the act and up until the repeal of prohibition were extremely strict also.
17 Tariff Act of 1930: § 1305. Accessed 31/07/18.
18 It is on the basis of scientific merit that the ban on contraceptive goods would later be challenged in *United States v One Package of Japanese Pessaries 1936*.
19 Robert Spoo, *Without Copyright: Piracy, Publishing, and the Public Domain*, (Oxford: Oxford University Press, 2013), p. 159.
20 Quoted in Ibid. p. 171.
21 Ibid. p. 168.
22 Among the signees was Lawrence whose text *Lady Chatterley's Lover* would be pirated by Roth in 1930, for which he would later be jailed on charges of distributing obscenity.
23 Ibid. p. 155.
24 *United States v Ulysses*, p. 74.
25 Ibid. p. 98.
26 It was in fear of potential prosecution that both Viking Press in the United States and Faber and Faber in the United Kingdom declined to publish the text.
27 Ibid. p. 99.
28 Ibid. p. 299.

29 Ronell, *Crack Wars*, p. 29.
30 The double meaning of immunity is here at play: in one sense, it signals the absence of any legitimate legal violence to be forced upon the subject or text. In another, more pharmacological sense, it is also the process whereby the foreign body is prevented from corrupting the healthy body. By figuring the text as immune from the accusation of obscenity, an insertion into the inside from the outside is required, but done in the name of protecting the interior from a more dangerous threat. We can see here a shift from the how the previous trials figured the text: in those trials, the text itself was the foreign body corrupting the national body; here, the body of the text is being figured as neutral, immune from this accusation of potential corruptive influence. Later, in the *Lady Chatterley* trial, a further pharmacological transformation will occur, wherein the text will be figured as the cure, and the national body will be figured as needing the intervention of the *pharmakon* to prevent further corruption.
31 Ibid. p. 120.
32 Ibid. p. 122.
33 Ibid. p. 125.
34 Ibid. p. 126.
35 Ibid. p. 128.
36 Dos Passos, as Woolsey will later, justifies the truth value of *Ulysses* through the introduction of another medium, the image. Once again, the truth of the text necessitates the introduction of a foreign and exterior substance in order to speak its truth, belying the truth being spoken and hinting at the presence of untruth being deferred through the act of speaking its truth.
37 This tactic has another purpose: it would be difficult for the defence to posit the figure of the average reader and describe his response to the text if there were in fact readers present who could dissent to their claims about this normative representative of their interpretations. It is much easier to figure a norm in the absence of that which it purports to represent.
38 Ibid. p. 175.
39 Ibid. p. 238.
40 There is a tension here in the figuring of Joyce as a solitary figure. In figuring Joyce's value as deriving from his distance from the people and the market, which will be figured as a marker of the people's will, a certain contempt for the people is thus evident in Ernst's argumentation.
41 Ibid. p. 239.
42 The specific function of the citation will be explored more thoroughly in the following chapter wherein a citation can effectively replace its author.
43 Ibid. p. 231.
44 In this sense, what we have here is the obverse of Edelman's reproductive futurism, a fantasy not of the future but of a past. And indeed, for the fantasy of reproductive futurism to take place, this imagined shared past must also be in place. In the next chapter, I will explore this fantasy formation of an idyllic and shared past under threat as it occurs in the criticism of T.S. Eliot and F.R. Leavis.
45 Ibid. p. 244.
46 Ibid. p. 244.
47 Ibid. p. 245.
48 Ibid. pp. 247–248.
49 Ibid. p. 249.
50 Ibid. pp. 249–250.
51 Ibid. p. 251.–
52 Ibid. p. 255.
53 Ibid.
54 Ibid. p. 232.
55 Ibid. p. 259.
56 Ibid. p. 180.

57 Ibid. p. 260.
58 Ibid. p. 263.
59 Ibid. p. 309.
60 Ibid. pp. 309–310.
61 Ibid. p. 310.
62 Ibid.
63 Ibid.
64 Ibid.
65 Ibid.
66 Ibid. pp. 310–311.
67 Ibid. p. 311.
68 Wolfgang Streit, *Joyce/Foucault: Sexual Confessions*, (London: University of Michigan Press, 2004), p. 143.
69 *United States v Ulysses*, p. 312.
70 Streit, *Joyce/Foucault*, p. 142.
71 *United States vs Ulysses*, p. 312.
72 Ibid.
73 Ibid.
74 Streit, *Joyce/Foucault*, p. 141.
75 *United States v Ulysses*, p. 314.

Bibliography

Bataille, Georges, *The Accursed Share, An Essay on General Economy, Volume One: Consumption*, (New York: Zone Books 1991).

Bell, Daniel, *The Cultural Contradictions of Capitalism*, (New York: Basic Books, 1996).

Gramsci, Antonio, 'America and Fordism', in *The Gramsci Reader: Selected Writings 1916–1935*, (New York: New York University Press, 2000), pp. 275–300.

Van Hulle, Dirk, *James Joyce's 'Work in Progress': Pre-book Publications of Finnegans Wake Fragments*, (London: Routledge, 2016).

Lerner, Michael, *Dry Manhattan: Prohibition in New York City*, (London: Harvard University Press, 2011).

Moscato, Michael and Leslie LeBlanc, *The United States Vs One Book Called Ulysses by James Joyce: Documents and Commentary- A Fifty Year Perspective*, (Frederick, MD: University Publications of America, 1984).

Potter, Rachel, *Obscene Modernism: Literary Censorship and Experiment 1900–1940*, (Oxford: Oxford University Press, 2013).

Ronell, Avital, *Crack Wars: Literature Adiction, Mania*, (London: University of Illinois Press, 2004).

Spoo, Robert, *Without Copyright: Piracy, Publishing, and the Public Domain*, (Oxford: Oxford University Press, 2013).

Streit, Wolfgang, *Joyce/Foucault: Sexual Confessions*, (London: University of Michigan Press, 2004).

Wittenmyer, Anne, *The History of the Woman's Temperance Crusade*, (Boston, MA: James Earle, 1882).

4

THE TRIUMPH OF 'LIFE'

In *Homo Sacer*, Giorgio Agamben distinguishes between two forms of life as described in Aristotle, *bios* and *zoe*. *Bios*, Agamben argues represents 'the form or way of living proper to an individual or group', whereas *zoe* names 'the simple fact of living as such'.[1] As a form of living, *bios* is the means by which a set of subjects assume a collective name and identity: it is under that collective name that each individual subject is given a name that places them in a particular relation to the collective. *Bios* is a name for civic life, it names the ends and values to which subjects in a set are to work towards and co-ordinate their desire around. *Zoe* then comes to name that part of life that cannot be subsumed by *bios*, a remainder Agamben terms 'bare life'.[2] *Bios* depends upon bare life for its very existence; without individual life, a social link between bodies cannot be formed. But bare life also stands as a reminder of the arbitrariness of the civic code. *Bios* can never claim precedence over *zoe* as long as it is seen to be dependent upon it. As such, an exclusion of bare life must be substantiated by *bios*, an exclusion that can never be completed because of the above-mentioned dependency. *Zoe* is included in *bios* through the means of exclusion whereby that which comes to represent bare life is prohibited in the name of the protection of the civic. This relation between the inclusion and exclusion is the founding operation of politics, Agamben argues, with politics being 'the place in which life [has] to transform itself into good life and in which what had to be politicized were always already bare life'.[3] Law, in this schema, is the means by which this transformation occurs: in the legal decision, the distinction between *bios* and *zoe* is made. The function of law, according to Agamben, has always been the management of life, the demarcation of good and evil forms of living. In a more psychoanalytic register, I wish to use, but also trouble, this definition by adding another dimension between the two forms of life: both *bios* and *zoe* bring with them two forms of enjoyment. Understood this way, the law also has not only the role of distinguishing between forms

DOI: 10.4324/9781003202509-4

of life but also regulating the forms of enjoyment that are concomitant with the good life and bare life.[4]

Agamben's distinction is useful for thinking about the way in which the obscene is figured in legal trials as it coincides with the 19th-century's interest in the forms of enjoyment that the literary text elicits in subjects. Good literature is that which is on the side of culture and civic virtues, whilst pornography instigates a form of enjoyment felt to be harmful to the public body. The distinction Agamben defines is then operative in obscenity law. But, as I have also argued, the boundaries between the literary and the obscene are more fluid than the law's distinction allows for; so too for Agamben's distinction between *bios* and *zoe*. For Agamben, the distinction is troubled in the figure of the sovereign. The sovereign is the one who decides the exception and, as such, is both inside and outside the law: the sovereign is both the representative of the law's stability and a signifier of its contingency. It is with the figure of the sovereign and his double, *homo sacer*, that the paradox of sovereignty is made manifest.[5] However, I wish to complicate this manoeuvre: for Agamben, it is in these particular signifiers, the sovereign and *homo sacer*, that the distinction between *bios* and *zoe* is troubled. But it is also how it is solved, their function as doubles of each other maintain each other's place and the stability of the law. This problematic, I wish to argue, is not locatable in certain signifiers but in signification as such. If the instance of speech produces a split between the subject of the enunciation and the enunciating subject, then in every speech act a split between the subject and the symbolic order is made, that is between bare life and the polis. Two problems with Agamben's prognosis emerge here: first, it becomes very hard to distinguish between *zoe* and *bios* at any given time when the signifier is given the role of representing that distinction: in the act of distinction, the split between the concepts is troubled once again. Second, the agency of the signifier attests to another form of life operative in Agamben's dynamic, the life of the signifier itself: the signifier has a life of its own, it means otherwise in spite of the living subject's intentions. But to call this agency life is to trouble Agamben's schema because bare life is the condition of possibility for *bios*. The signifier cannot be said to live in this manner, but instead, it would be a form of living death, underwriting life itself. Life, as it were, is underwritten by death, and the signifier is both the mediator and the condition of this dynamic. In my previous chapter, this living death of the signifier has been discussed under the name of the death drive. In this chapter, the indistinguishability between the force of life and the work of the death drive operative in sexuality will become more apparent.

This again draws us back to the work of Lawrence and the key problems his fictions confront. Much of his fiction explores the problem of the signifier and the desire to find a form of life beyond it. This interest very quickly transforms into an experience of anxiety in the face of death. The investment in life very quickly becomes a fascination with death in Lawrence. How then does Lawrence become a champion of a criticism that conceives of life as a universally positive attribute and sees Lawrence as the champion of the good life, *bios*, and the law? In short, my answer will be that the forms of criticism that emerge after the author's death and are utilized throughout the *Lady Chatterley* trial constitute a repression of precisely this deathly aspect of Lawrence's writing.

The 1960 trial establishes an even greater convergence between the law and literary criticism than demonstrated in any other of the trials in this book. This chapter will trace the reading practices operative in the trial and in the criticism of F.R. Leavis, analysing the necessary omissions and repressions operative in both witness testimonies and in readings of Lawrence's texts in order to make *Lady Chatterley* a signifier of health and life. In doing so, the trial also maintains the distinction between forms of enjoyment, distinctions that both the law and literary criticism help to maintain.

The 1960 trial of D.H. Lawrence's novel *Lady Chatterley's Lover* was the first major test of the newly created legislation for the policing of obscenity in the United Kingdom. The Obscene Publication Act 1959 differed substantially from the previous legislation. The new statute came about as a result of successful lobbying from The Society of Authors in response to the then Conservative Home Secretary Sir David Maxwell Fyfe's decision to prosecute five novels in 1954.[6] The union demanded substantial protections for the literary text against accusations of pornography. At the Parliamentary Select Committee, the Chairman of the SOA, Sir Allen Herbert, made the argument that the Hicklin Test's criteria could not distinguish between the respectable literary author and the obscene pornographer:

> It is the other man you want to get after, the man who sits down and thinks 'I want to make my readers as randy as I can, as often as I can'. That is the man you are after. He is not bothering whether he is corrupting anybody. He is frankly marketing lust, he is marketing something he knows he can sell. The problem you have to face is to distinguish [...] between myself and the other fellow.[7]

Herbert here pleas for a distinction between literature and pornography that the Hicklin test is designed to ignore the intention of the author when composing the text. The distinction between the author and the pornographer is dependent upon a full acceptance of the necessity of obscenity legislation. In order to move the problem of obscenity away from the signifier itself and onto the subject, Herbert has to situate the presence of obscene enjoyment in the domain of the other. This other man's enjoyment is depicted as a perverse enjoyment in eliciting the reader's desire, in manipulating their body. It is also absent of any economy or propriety, and it has no set limit to its enjoyment. It is also apparent that the enjoyment of the pornographic other comes at the expense of the respectable author's enjoyment: an economy of enjoyment is set up between the author and 'the other fellow' in which the author is found to be in deficit. The law itself is not understood to be the marker of this loss; instead, it is this fantasized other who is the cause of the legitimate author's lack. The other who won't play by the rules and enjoys too much is the cause of the difficulty the union members' discontent. The perverse enjoyment is not located in language itself but can in fact be located in the author's intention or the effect on the reader. Language is thus left untainted by obscenity and literature's value in comparison to pornography consists of the absence of enjoyment. Key to this argument is the evacuation of any enjoyment from the signifier. The law's function, according to this argument, is the maintenance, or, in a more biopolitical register, the continued immunization of the signifier from this unhealthy enjoyment.

The pornographer is also figured as a man who enters into the market with an affect and not an object. This appearance on the market of lust would seem to signify a perverse relation to the market, but at the same time, by virtue of the pornographer's knowledge that lust sells, the market continues to function despite this apparent perverse affect entering into the economy. Or perhaps, it is the market itself that comes under suspicion of obscenity in its capacity to disseminate texts to whomever desires them. But this would ignore the author's very dependency upon the market to disseminate his own works to the public and receive an income for his endeavours. And if the author is also enmeshed in the same economy as the pornographer, it is also not clear what object or affect the literary author brings to the market that distinguishes his wares from that of the pornographer.

A definition of the literary text and the obscene text are absent from this description, and the ambiguity of the signified and the problem of the interpretation of the text are elided in favour of the designation of a character type based not upon the text produced, but the form of the writer's enjoyment. From a reading of the text in isolation, free from a knowledge of the writer's intentions, as has been demonstrated in the previous chapters, it is impossible to fully distinguish between the literary and the obscene, the two categories can be said to describe the same text. Thus, the author and his desire are introduced as a fantasmatic supplement in order to make this distinction possible.

It is towards a greater distinction between art and pornography, between good and bad *jouissance*, that the 1959 Act was designed. The criteria for obscenity are expanded from the previous definition:

> an article shall be deemed to be obscene if its effect or [...] if taken as a whole, such as to tend to deprave and corrupt persons who are likely, having regard to all relevant circumstances, to read, see or hear the matter contained or embodied in it.[8]

The two major additions here are the condition that the text must now be considered as a whole and the introduction of a 'likely' reader rather than the previous legislation's emphasis on the 'vulnerable' reader. These two changes add a degree of context with which defence councils can argue. No longer does a single section of a text, taken in isolation from the larger context of the novel or poem, become liable for the banning of the entire piece. As such, the defence can now argue that any potentially obscene passages are only meaningful in relation to other passages. The emphasis on a likely reader also places the burden on the prosecution to credibly prove that the text will find its way to a vulnerable reader capable of being depraved and corrupted by the text in question. As this chapter will demonstrate, these two changes offer the defence council for Penguin Books more nuanced strategies for defending a text than was afforded by the previous legislation.

In the following section of the act, a further mitigating circumstance is added to distinguish between art and pornography, the category of 'public good':

> (1) A person shall not be convicted of an offence against section two of this Act, and an order for forfeiture shall not be made under the foregoing section, if it is proved that publication of the article in question is justified as being for the public good on the ground that it is in the interests of science, literature, art or learning, or of other objects of general concern.
>
> (2) It is hereby declared that the opinion of experts as to the literary, artistic, scientific or other merits of an article may be admitted in any proceedings under this Act either to establish or to negative the said ground.[9]

This defence allows for a distinction between art and pornography on the grounds of literary merit. Thus, a text can be said to contain obscene material but, by virtue of its literariness, cannot be considered obscene under the statute. Again, the distinction here is between *bios* and *zoe*, two forms of enjoyment: the civic and constructive enjoyment implied by the term public good is therefore a legitimate response to the text, whereas a form of enjoyment that is private and against the forms of knowledge defined in the act. The disciplines of 'science, literature, art and learning' are figured as being able to co-opt the sexual into their bodies of knowledge without being corrupted or corrupting to the subject who practises them. However, sexuality, in its pornographic form, is figured as outside and as threatening these bodies of knowledge. As the second article makes clear, it is the role of an expert witness, a master of their discourse, to adjudicate what form of enjoyment a text is depicting or advocating. In the case of *Lady Chatterley*, the prominent discourse used by the defence was the discourse of literary criticism.

Here, it is important to note the marked change of status the works of Lawrence had undergone within literary criticism between the initial publication of *Lady Chatterley's Lover* in 1928 and the date of the obscenity trial in 1960. The novel was officially banned in the United Kingdom without trial. Contemporaneous reviews of the novel in England were particularly vitriolic. A review in *John Bull* serves as an extreme but not uncommon reaction. In this review, Lawrence is compared to 'lascivious [...] oriental writers', and the novel itself is described as 'the most evil outpouring that has ever besmirched the literature in our country'.[10] The text is linked to a threatening foreign realm as is often the case in depictions of obscenity, this time France: 'The sewers of French pornography would be dragged in vain to find a parallel in beastliness. The creations of muddy-minded perverts, peddled in the back-street bookstalls of Paris are prudish by comparison'.[11] These attempts to link obscenity to a foreign otherness recall the parallels drawn between *The Rainbow* and Zola and *Women in Love* to German philosophy. The obscene is that which does not belong in England, and in the care of *Lady Chatterley's Lover*, it does not even belong in Paris. The text by virtue of its obscenity is designated no proper place, outside the Symbolic and in the realm of abject bare life. This association between sexual transgression and exile is extended to the author himself: 'Mr Lawrence has a diseased mind. He is obsessed with sex and we have no doubt that he will be ostracized by all except the most degenerate coteries of the world'.[12] Here again, the obscene is relegated to the exterior of the world, denied a nation. As too is the author as representative of the obscene. The article performs a strategy of removing the proper place for this enjoyment, declaring it unfit for France or the tainted orient, instead delegating the author himself as the source of obscenity. This strategy of locating the degeneracy of the text in Lawrence himself is repeated in the assertion that the text 'was created [...] out of the turgid vigour of a poisoned genius'.[13] One can also note the enjoyment operative in the act of denunciation, that same 'turgid vigour', which the review declares to be repellent, is fully visible in the repeated gestures of disgust, returning every few lines to state the reviewers disgust in ever increasing extremes. The signifier is again found inadequate to coincide with the full meaning of the sexual. The same economy of the pornographer defined by Herbert is operative in the act of policing him, suggesting a reciprocity of enjoyment between the pornographer and the censor.

If the 1959 Act was designed to differentiate between the respectable author and the perverse pornographer, as Herbert describes it, then the example of Lawrence troubles this distinction: it is precisely as the obscene and threatening figure of the pornographer that Lawrence is perceived as during his lifetime and the years immediately following his death. These accusations and responses to his work will form the majority of the prosecution's case against *Lady Chatterley* in 1960.

During the 1940s and 1950s, however, the reputation of Lawrence within literary criticism markedly changed. A major catalyst for this radical shift in perception was the work of F.R. Leavis, particularly his book-length study *D.H. Lawrence: Novelist*. The results of Leavis's work on Lawrence were transformative not only of the reception of Lawrence within the institution of the university but also, as Sean Matthews argues, the very discourse itself:

> As a result of his championing of Lawrence, there [was] renewed attention to the Eastwood writer's provincial, working class origins, and to the distinctive voice and concerns of his literary achievement. This work formed a wider reassessment of the nature and methods of literary criticism [...].[14]

The Leavis project is one specifically formulated to re-evaluate the values and hierarchies of previous criticism.[15] Lawrence, by virtue of being both working class and accused of obscenity, becomes emblematic of this project. It is towards a transformation of Lawrence's texts from that of the pornographer to a literary artist that Leavis is concerned with. Leavis, in *D.H. Lawrence*, claims that his aim is 'to win clear recognition for the nature of Lawrence's greatness'.[16] The use of the word 'win' implies an antagonistic relationship to previous critics including those whom Leavis elsewhere acknowledges as precursors to his project. Key among these influences was T.S. Eliot, who had on a number of occasions made disparaging remarks about Lawrence. Leavis agrees with Eliot's assessment that the critic's function should be 'the common pursuit of true judgement' and, as such, commits to the belief that the discourse of literary criticism is a discourse of truth, in which the true meaning of a text can be known and reported.[17] But, as I have noted elsewhere in previous chapters in regard to both the work of Matthew Arnold and T.S. Eliot, these discourses of truth ground themselves upon certain empty signifiers continually referring back to themselves in order to justify the hierarchies and values they declare. For Eliot, one such signifier was 'tradition', and it is this term that Leavis appropriates throughout his work, but of particular interest here is its function in *D.H. Lawrence* and *The Great Tradition*. In Leavis's work, there is a modification of Eliot's strategy, and it is linked to the introduction of a working-class author into the tradition: Lawrence himself derives from the 'living tradition' of the working class.[18]

The term 'living tradition' appears in Eliot's criticism. In *After Strange Gods*, Eliot defines a living tradition as 'all those habitual actions, habits, and customs, from the most significant religious rite to our conventional way of greeting a stranger, which represent the blood kinship of "the same people living in the same place"'.[19] Tradition here is understood as a composite of signifiers and their related signifieds. This matrix of signifiers is given a representative function, and it stands in place of and defines the subjects that perform it. But this representative function requires recourse to the very tradition that Eliot is trying to define, whereby Bloom's definition of a nation in *Ulysses* comes to signify the final definition of a tradition's meaning.[20] The definition of tradition here effects a feedback loop, whereby its definition is dependent upon its own terms, a performative strategy that produces the essences upon which it depends. For Eliot, James Joyce represents the orthodox aspects of the Christian tradition, whereas Lawrence embodies a heretical relation to tradition and as such cannot be incorporated.

To say a tradition is living, for Eliot, names a temporal quality of its being: the fact that it continues to exist. Tradition's relation to life does not affect its status as tradition, other traditions have existed in the past and others will emerge in the future. Therein lies the shift of focus in the criticism of F.R. Leavis. The strategy by which to incorporate Lawrence into the tradition of literature depends upon the introduction of the empty signifier 'Life', into literary criticism whereby a text's relation to life signifies its value as literature. In *The Great Tradition*, Leavis argues that what distinguishes Jane Austen, George Eliot, Henry James and Joseph Conrad from the rest of English writers is

> an intense focus, an unusually developed interest in life. For far from having anything of Flaubert's disgust or disdain or boredom, they are all distinguished by a vital capacity for experience, a kind of reverent openness before life, and a marked moral intensity.[21]

The writer must be interested in life and be reverently open to it. Life, here, is not a quality of an object under observation as in Eliot but is now an ontological category that the author must adopt a position towards, either for or against. The political dimension of this distinction is clear. It effects a clear demarcation between those on the side of life and those on the side of death.[22] This relation is specifically figured as moral: the author's relationship to life determines his/her moral quality, and this moral quality admits or disqualifies the texts from the tradition. It is interesting, then, to note that Flaubert does not qualify for introduction because of his 'disgust', 'disdain' and 'boredom'. These qualities are presented as antithetical to life, and following the logic of Leavis's argument, therefore, mark out Flaubert as an immoral writer. That Flaubert is French and the other authors are English and American is important because it figures one of France's canonical authors as an enemy of life. A parochial nationalism is at work within this form of criticism which would set the living tradition of English literature against the life denying aesthetes of Europe. This is another difference from Eliot's use of tradition which was cosmopolitan if decidedly Eurocentric. Leavis's moralistic English nationalism is structured in the same way as the earlier critical responses to Lawrence, wherein obscenity is linked to various foreign nations, the difference being that Lawrence himself is now found on the side of life.[23]

Leavis's critique of Flaubert is itself a wholesale appropriation of Lawrence's assessment that Flaubert 'stood away from life as from a leprosy'.[24] Lawrence's writing functions here as the source of Leavis's critical valuations. In *D.H. Lawrence*, Leavis bestows upon Lawrence's oeuvre a privilege he does not extend to other authors, even those of *The Great Tradition*: '[Lawrence] educates for the kind of criticism that here and there it challenges- it provides the incitement and the criteria'.[25] Lawrence's texts are here figured as an explicit challenge to and refusal of previous forms of criticism that had dismissed him as either obscene or non-literary. It also, following this argument, provides the groundwork for a new criticism and a new understanding of itself. As such, Lawrence's texts in their apparent originality provide Leavis with texts that '[create] the concepts with which they are concerned'.[26] Thus, close reading and the use of large quotations of a text are used in Leavis's work on Lawrence as a demonstration of the text's self-sufficiency, what Leavis terms its 'organic wholeness'.[27] But as to why Lawrence is afforded this privilege and the other authors in the tradition, his supposed precursors, are not, remains unclear. Furthermore, as has been demonstrated in Leavis's wholesale appropriation of Lawrence's terminology, to define both those texts that belong in the tradition and those that do not, the criteria that are offered by Lawrence's writing also come to define all previous works. *The Great Tradition*, beginning with Austen and culminating in Lawrence, is constructed by Leavis retrospectively in order to claim legitimacy for Lawrence's work as literature. The texts that go into constructing a narrative of a tradition are then only so many symptoms of an initial investment. The investment is held in place by the master signifier 'Life', functioning as the ground upon which this initial investment can stake its claim to truth and thus repress its fantasmatic elements. As discussed in the previous chapter in the case of the discourse of drugs, in order for enjoyment to be considered legitimate, it must be grounded in truth: the master signifier 'life' can thus function as a way to ground the critic's enjoyment in truth, the critic's *jouissance* is transfigured into a palatable desire for truth and thus on the side of bios and the polis.

Both Leavis and Eliot's dependency upon citation as the last instance is symptomatic of the malleability, or the duplicity, of the signifier: in these instances, the signifier has the capacity to end an argument, to say *more than* enough, and thus not need to be explained. The use of citation introduces a circular logic, wherein the truth claim is founded upon its own self-evidence. But, if it was self-evident, it would not need to be cited, thus rendering the act of citation superfluous to its aim of revealing what is already revealed. In this excess, there is also evidence that the signifier does too little. The act of repetition indicates an insufficiency of the truth being claimed to evidence itself; the truth is dependent upon the signifier to represent its veracity, and in repetition, the signifier shows its incompatibility with its task of truth telling. In his essay 'Signature, Event, Context', Derrida explains this ambiguous quality of citation:

> Every sign, linguistic or nonlinguistic, spoken or written [...] in a small or large unit, can be cited, put between quotation marks; in so doing it can break with every given context, engendering an infinity of new contexts in a manner which is absolutely illimitable. This does not imply that the mark is valid outside of a context, but on the contrary that there are only contexts without any center or absolute anchoring [ancrage]. This citationality, this duplication or duplicity, this iterability of the mark is neither an accident nor an anomaly, it is that (normal/abnormal) without which a mark could not even have a function called "normal".[28]

Citation involves the moving of the text out of one context and placing into another. Each context confers meaning upon the given quotation, and it enters into a different metonymic chain in which the previous and subsequent signifiers alter the way in which the citation can be interpreted. To take Eliot's citation of Joyce as an example, it becomes clear that in Eliot's usage, the reference to Bloom's definition of nation as 'the same people living in the same place' serves to ground his definition of tradition and thus continues to decide which texts constitute orthodoxy and which constitute heterodoxy. The citation in Eliot is thus the basis for the formation of knowledge. But in Joyce's text, the very same sentence actually serves to disrupt the formation of knowledge in relation to the discussion on Irish nationhood, as we can gather from the hostility with which those around him receive it with. The signifier does not change but the context radically conditions the function of the words in relation to truth.[29] The very fact that this is possible is evidence of the signifier's 'duplicity', its inability to ground itself outside of the metonymic chain. The citability of the signifier is precisely what allows language to function as such: the absence of a norm in relation to the signifier, the inability to fully correspond with its referent, is the norm of language. Citability allows for repetition of the signifier within new contexts and produces the infinity of new contexts and meanings.

What I wish to show here is the groundlessness of Eliot and Leavis's claims to truth, their dependence on eliding the ambiguity of language that their arguments depend upon. But to argue, only this point would itself elide a certain historical fact: these truth statements did and still do function as anchors upon which the discourse of literary criticism functions. I would like to posit the reason for the perceived validity of the truth claims of Eliot and Leavis as the position from which they speak and the structure of their discourse. The production of knowledge is intricately linked to the dissemination of power, and it is power, I wish to argue, that fixes the signifier in place and declares certain claims as false and certain untrue. But this, the claim to truth from the position of power, is not enough to reproduce the effect of truth. Geoff Bucher elucidates on this point when he argues that '[k]nowledge is not immediately power [...] – it is real because the subject believes it is authorized by convention'.[30] What is required for a truth claim to become knowledge is the production of a subject who desires to believe this claim. The instability of the claim to truth that Derrida delineates not only provides the impossibility of grounding the truth claim but also demonstrates that the groundlessness of the demand is also the source of its power in that it produces a reader who is willing not only to believe the claim but also one who is willing to place the burden of proof on themselves and not the master. What presents itself here is a relation between the teacher and his student between the discourse of the master and the discourse of the university.

The trial enacts these tensions between the literary text and truth, the ambiguity of the citation, and between the master and his student. I will focus on three episodes during the trial which best demonstrate these tensions. First, I will examine the expert testimony of Richard Hoggart whose testimony at the trial was deemed vital in legitimizing Lawrence's writing as authentically working class. Second, I shall explore the unspoken witness proof of T.S. Eliot in order to analyse the anxieties that his proof elicited from the defence. Finally, I shall turn to the use of the discourse of psychiatry in the trial and the way in which the defence focused on sexuality as a positive and healthy force, a formulation I aim to problematize. Similarly, to the 1933 *Ulysses* trial, what is at stake in this trial is the immunization of literature, the removal of a perceived absence of truth, non-being and death. If Woolsey's decision made the literary text a medicine, The *Lady Chatterley* trial makes the text a form of therapy: Lawrence changes from the corrupting pornographer into the prophet of sexual health.

As mentioned previously, due to the changes in the statute, the value of witness testimony in the *Lady Chatterley* trial far outweighs the importance placed on witnesses in previous trials. As such, it is worth briefly discussing the political dimension of this shift. The function and duty of a witness at a trial is, in effect, to convey the truth to the court. The truth is taken as a property that can be perceived universally and described through language. However, the value of witness testimony consists in the individual subject's relation to and specific figuration of the truth. Shoshana Felman discusses this tension in her text *Testimony*:

> Since the testimony cannot be simply relayed, repeated, or reported by another without thereby losing its function as testimony, the burden of the witness- in spite of his or her alignment with other witnesses- is a radically unique, noninterchangeable, and solitary burden.[31]

The sole value of testimony is predicated on the subject's 'unique' and 'noninterchangeable' relation to the event that she is asked to tell. It is then premised on the eradication of the other from the subject's discourse. This noninterchangeability has two dimensions that complicate the function of testimony in legal proceedings. First, the fact that testimony precludes exchange means that it cannot enter into an economy of truth claims made by other witnesses. A trial can be interpreted as an exchange and valuation of differing truth claims, an exchange predicated upon the value of testimony. The uniqueness of the subject's relation to the truth thus renders this relation untranslatable. Which brings us to the second complication of the noninterchangeability of the witness's testimony, its relation to the signifier. Signification in predicated on the exchange of signifiers, standing in for the subject and her relation to the truth. Testimony is addressed to the other in order to differentiate the speaking subject from the other itself and in so differentiating itself attains its value and its truth. However, this address must be done in both the dimension of the other, in this case, the courtroom, and through the other's language. True testimony is then an impossible demand.[32]

The demand to tell the truth, the incitement to discourse, allows for this deadlock to be bypassed. As Felman argues:

> [T]he *appointment* to bear witness is, paradoxically enough, an appointment to transgress the confines of that isolated stance, to speak for and to others. [...] [T]he witness's speech is one which, by its very definition, transcends the witness who is but its medium, the medium of realization of the testimony. [...] By virtue of the fact that the testimony is *addressed* to others, the witness, from within the solitude of his own stance is the vehicle of an occurrence, a reality, a stance or a dimension *beyond* himself.[33]

As Felman alludes to here, the act of testimony takes place in the domain of the Other, that is, to others and through the language of the other. As such, the impossibility of true testimony is bypassed because it becomes the witness's duty not so much to speak their truth but to be the conduit through which a predetermined and prescripted truth is spoken. In basic terms, the witness is selected by either the prosecution or defence to speak a certain truth that befits the narrative being offered; witnesses are routinely briefed and coached by their council in order to maintain a stance that is commensurate with the position given by other witnesses. The choice of witnesses opens up a politics of representation, wherein the representatives for certain peoples or disciplines are chosen not so much to speak their own truth but rather to speak a truth appropriate to the norm that governs the discourse in which they speak. To take social class as an example, only certain individuals are chosen by power to represent the working class. Their selection is not based upon the proximity of themselves to the truth or authenticity of their class but their ability to suit the purposes certain narratives of social class that are beneficial to power.

This politics of representation operative in the trial mirrors those previously noted in Leavis's canon building. Working-class voices are admitted into the canon, offering opportunities and privileges to those who had previously been silenced. This admission however has certain stipulations: Lawrence's admission into the canon is predicated on the maintenance of the canon itself. Those aspects of Lawrence that were before heterogeneous and threatening to the values of literary criticism are elided in place of a reading of Lawrence that emphasizes both his Englishness, a commitment to life and his advocation of socially acceptable institutions, in the case of the trial and *Lady Chatterley's Lover* itself, the institution of heterosexual marriage. Lawrence's role as representative of the working class does not then represent the wholesale entry of working-class voices into the discourse of literature, but rather functions as a prefigured conception of how the working class should be and write like. Lawrence then functions not as a representative of the multitude of voices but a carefully selected and managed example that excludes as much as it invites.

It is in this context that the testimony of Richard Hoggart during the trial takes on special importance. Of working-class origins himself, Hoggart's function in the trial was to argue from a position of personal experience the culture of the working class for whom Lawrence was being made to figure. His presence at the trial was also predicated on his text *The Uses of Literacy* published two years before the trial. In this text, Hoggart analyses the effect of newly emergent mass media of working-class communities, particularly those in his native Leeds. He begins the text with condemnation of the way in which the working class have been represented in the past but also with reservations about precisely the valorization of working-class culture I have noted in Leavis:

> No doubt such an over-emphasis is often inspired by a strong admiration for the potentialities of working-class people and a consequent pity for their situation. Related to it is a more positive over-expectation which one frequently finds among middle-class intellectuals with strong social consciences.[34]

Hoggart is wary of any overdetermination of the potentialities of working-class cultures either as a threat to civic life or as its potential saviour. He is also careful to note that his personal experiences could lead him to a similar overvaluation, or as he puts it, 'nostalgia [...] colouring the material in advance'.[35] This nostalgia, I wish to argue, is what links Hoggart's politics to Leavis's despite his own reservations. Nostalgia in this sense does not indicate a relation to the material world or to lived experience: both Hoggart and Leavis grew up in very different cultures. Rather, I wish to argue that their shared nostalgia is founded upon a shared relationship to language and its perceived function of mimesis.

Hoggart argues that literature, specifically the work of Lawrence, 'may bring us really close to the quality of working-class life'.[36] The work of literature then functions as a witness to a culture, a testimony that can be understood by other subjects outside those cultures. The value of the work of literature lies in the validity of its representation of life. In contrast to the true literary text, Hoggart identifies the endless rain of 'confetti-literature' produced by a growing mass culture.[37] Mass culture, according to Hoggart, threatens the identities of working-class cultures through homogenization: 'the remnants of what was at least in parts an urban culture "of the people" are being destroyed [...] [and] the new mass culture is in some important ways less healthy than the often crude culture it is replacing'.[38] The recourse to health reveals an important aspect of Hoggart's critique of consumer culture; these cultures, however 'crude', are the vestiges of life, and it is this life that is under threat from market forces that are implicitly linked to death. By extension, the literary work that represented these cultures so truthfully is on the side of life, whereas the commodities available for purchase are figured as a threat to the literary work and to life itself. We have then a reproduction of the structure of Herbert's argument against the pornographer, whereby the literary is positioned as a form of healthy enjoyment, and market forces are implicated in a form of enjoyment that is destructive.[39]

> Later in the text, Hoggart cites Lawrence in his condemnation of mass culture:
>
> Most mass-entertainments are in the end what D. H. Lawrence described as 'anti-life'. They are full of a corrupt brightness, of improper appeals and moral evasions. To recall instances: they tend towards a view of the world in which progress is conceived as a seeking of material possessions, equality as a moral levelling, and freedom as the ground for endless irresponsible pleasure.[40]

As noted above, in regard to Eliot and Leavis, the grounds for this form of argumentation are again a citation from a literary text. Lawrence, once again, functions as the source of the veracity of the analysis of mass culture and once again what exactly is meant by life goes unsaid. A clue is perhaps given in the effects of mass culture, specifically the accusation that the market promotes 'endless irresponsible pleasure'. Once again, the market is accused of facilitating anarchic and destructive enjoyment. That this pleasure is described as endless alludes to the absence of a goal or stable object towards which this pleasure is aimed: what is improper about this enjoyment is that it has no proper place. Life is then perhaps the name for the flow of desire to its proper place, whilst death is figured here as a form of desire that loops back on itself, repeating itself and taking pleasure in this repetition.

But as previously mentioned, the operation of citation is ambiguous. The citation of Lawrence is here meant to ground the analysis in truth to connect the signifier to its proper place. However, citation implies repetition, the pulling of the signifier out of one context into another. In this way, the enjoyment brought about by the sovereign citation that fixes the signifier in its proper place, the enjoyment in truth, is dependent upon the same force, repetition, that is, the very symptom of the form of enjoyment that the truth is supposed to contrast against. The compulsion to repeat lies at the core of both reality and simulacrum, life and death: *bios* and *zoe* become undistinguishable.

But a distinction is required, and the literary text becomes the site upon which that distinction can and must be founded. The function of Hoggart's testimony as with many of the expert witnesses for the defence is to attest to the text being, in Lawrence's terms, an 'honest healthy book, necessary for today'.[41] The book, they would argue, was an attempt to convey a good and healthy relationship to sexuality from an authentic voice of the working class. In thus doing so, they could rebut the accusation of obscenity as elitist, prudish or both. This was the remit for Hoggart at the trial, the dimension beyond himself for which he gave testimony. Being working-class himself, Hoggart's function in regard to class in the trial was double: he and Lawrence were both representatives of the working class, and his function was to testify to the authenticity of his own position as working class. With this legitimacy, could he then legitimate the discourse of Lawrence as authentically working class. The manner in which this strategy is effected, that is through Hoggart's spoken testimony, highlights a series of tensions implicit in this claim to truth.

One of the main points of contestation in the trial was the perceived incongruity between literary merit and the obscene words used in the text. Referred to euphemistically as the 'four letter words' or the 'Anglo-Saxon' words during the trial, a strategy that both demonstrates these words' improper position within legal discourse but also in the case of 'Anglo-Saxon' provides a means by which to defend these words as inherently English in nature and relating to a past upon which a fantasy of wholeness can be projected.[42] The prosecution argued that Lawrence did not have to use these words and that his choice to use them was a clear indicator of both his perversity and his intention to illicit sexual feelings in the reader. The presence of these words was the means by which literature could be distinguished from pornography. The defence's retort to the accusation that these words were incommensurate with literary discourse was to appropriate the working class. These words, the argument went, were common parlance for a great many people in the nation, and their inclusion in the text was necessary for a sense of verisimilitude. It was upon this verisimilitude that the literary merit of Lawrence's text could be founded. Hoggart's improvised testimony on the matter of the obscenity in the everyday language of the working classes is instructive of the narrative the defence wished to produce in relation to the working class, the libidinal investments behind such a narrative and the necessary repression required to construct it. Upon cross examination by the prosecution, upon the necessity of using these words, Hoggart responded thusly:

> Fifty yards from this court this morning I heard a man say 'fuck' three times as he passed me. He was speaking to himself and he said 'fuck it, fuck it, fuck it' as he went past. If you have worked on a building site, as I have, you will find they recur over and over again. The man I heard this morning and the men on the building sites use these words as words of contempt, and one of the things Lawrence found most worrying about was the word for an important relationship had become a word of vile abuse. So one would say 'fuck you' to a man, although the thing has totally lost its meaning; it has simply become derision, and in this sense he wanted to re-establish the meaning of it, the proper use of it.[43]

The class dynamics present in this anecdote are complex and ambivalent. Hoggart as representative of the working classes bears witness to the truth of working-class discourse: the ubiquity of obscenity in everyday language. His status as working class, having worked on the building site and been among working-class culture, bestows upon his claim more veracity than that of a man of middle-class origins. The power of the truth claim is based upon Hoggart's proximity to working-class culture, his expertise as well as his lived experience. The anecdote implicitly demarcates two spaces, that of the court and that of the working classes '[f]ifty yards away'. The two spaces, seemingly small distances away from each other, are separated by their use of language, in this case the use of the word 'fuck'. The value of the anecdote and Hoggart as a representative of the working class is in collapsing the boundary between these two spaces: Hoggart cites the man on the street, bringing his obscene discourse into the courtroom from whence it had previously been repressed. It is by virtue of Hoggart's lived experience that he becomes the emissary of this obscene truth. Upon the legitimacy of Hoggart's origins is the verisimilitude of Lawrence's discourse justified and by extension the value of *Lady Chatterley's Lover* as a piece of literature.

But also operative in this statement is a strategy of distancing, whereby Hoggart asserts his separation from the working class. This separation is also the means by which the legitimacy of his testimony is guaranteed and the boundaries between the classes and their discourses are maintained. First, the initial positioning of Hoggart as an academic, an expert, distances him from the working classes. The social institution that confers upon him the status of expert is not that of the 'building site' but the university. It is the university that bestows his right to speak of being working class, only through this intermediary institution is the voice of the working class permitted into the court. Another act of distancing takes place in the anecdote itself: Hoggart appropriates the man's obscene discourse claiming it to be emblematic of working-class discourse as a whole, but nowhere in his statement does he claim to use that word; he has been present during its use but will not admit to using it. For as much as the obscenity of working-class discourse enters the courtroom from which it had previously been repressed, it does so here in the form of a citation and under the authority of an academic making a truth claim about persons who are not given the opportunity to bear witness for themselves. Thus, a repressive aspect of citationality appears, the appropriation of the working-class voice can function as a means to silence the voices of those it claims to represent. Representation of any authenticity is subsumed under the demands to present a pre-constructed norm. The citation is then put to work in order to ground this norm in truth held in place by power. Hoggart's testimony testifies to that dimension outside itself, the ambiguous politics of representation. Working-class voices are legitimized only under the terms specified by the pre-existing norm and between quotation marks.

Turning now to that norm and its purpose, there is a note of contempt in Hoggart's analysis of these everyday obscenities. What is at stake is 'the proper use' of these words. Rachel Bowlby, commenting on Hoggart's testimony, notes that 'the problem [for Hoggart] is not that the word names sex but that it does not'.[44] The working classes are using corrupted language and as such are corrupted themselves. The working class are thus depicted as both full of sexual life but also ignorant of the knowledge of it. The strategy of distancing I noted above here allows a form of immunization: Hoggart and his double, Lawrence, know the true meaning of these words and position themselves above the working class and removed from the taint of corruption. Lawrence's text then becomes a form of medicine for the working classes to purify their thoughts and allow them to speak properly. The literary text has changed from potential poison because of its indeterminacy into a cure due to its knowledge of the true meaning words: a new fantasy is being mapped onto the literary text by the defence.

As mentioned in relation to Leavis and Eliot, the fantasy being enunciated here by Hoggart and the other expert witnesses is dependent upon conceiving the site of truth, of life, and of sex, as being already lost. This loss of the site of truth at some point in the past situates the speaker as occupying a space after this loss has taken place. The speaker is thus afforded a privileged position that affords enjoyment by virtue of having access to the truth even in its degraded form. What is promised in this fantasy is a return to an imaginary state of wholeness in the future. The means by which that future is achieved is through repairing the two bearers of this perceived corruption: Language and Sex. The literary text is now appropriated for the production and protection of fantasy. But in order for this shift to take place, certain necessary repressions must take place, starting with the killing of the master and the emergence of the university.

In using these terms, I am drawing from Lacan's work on the four discourses in *Seminar XVII*. Lacan distinguishes between four discourses in this seminar:

the master, the university, the hysteric and the analyst. Each of these discourses is comprised of the same structure which Lacan designates as such:

$$\frac{\text{Agent}}{\text{Truth}} \rightarrow \frac{\text{Other}}{\text{Product}}$$

The agent of the discourse is the speaking being who addresses another speaking being, the arrow indicates the direction of the address, from agent to other, as well as the synchronic dimension of the production of discourse; it is in this direction that meaning is produced. This relation between the agent and its other also institutes power relations. Gérard Wajcman explains this dynamic as follows:

> Speech is addressed to another place in the direction of which it is delivered. Discourse as a signifying articulation establishes the social link that proceeds, from the place of speech as performance, to the place of speech as destination: to speak to an other is to act upon him. Thus discourse institutes power and conditions its exercise.[45]

To address another is to bring that person into language and into a certain context. It is, following Derrida, the citation of the other, the forcing of the other, through language, into a context decided by the agent of the discourse. The result is the binding of agent and other in a social link. The specific effect of the intervention of the agent upon the other is given in the bottom right corner of Lacan's schema. Finally, the bottom left quadrant indicates the truth operating through the agent and setting into motion the discourse. On the basis that the agent is not in control of the signifier, but instead, it is the signifier that defines the agent, the truth and the agent are separated. In Wacjman's terms, 'the agent suffers the truth rather than delivering it'.[46] The agent is as much a victim of citationality as the other whom he cites, in forging the social link with the other he speaks in the name of a truth separate from himself. In other words, the power structure initiated in the act of speaking does not confer this power onto the agent, he is not the owner of this power, and power speaks through the agent.

The first of Lacan's diagrams is the discourse of the master and the formula is arranged as such:

$$\frac{\mathbf{S^1}}{\mathbf{\$}} \rightarrow \frac{\mathbf{S^2}}{\boldsymbol{a}}$$

The type of discourse and thus, the specific power relations being produced is dependent upon which position the following mathemes are placed. These mathemes represent the constitutive parts of discourse and the order of their combination determines their effect. They are S^1, S^2, \$, and *a*. S^1 represents the master signifier and is placed in the role of agent. The master signifier, according to Lacan, 'holds the secret to knowledge'.[47] And it is around this secret that knowledge is formed: 'Knowledge initially arises at the moment at which S^1, comes to represent something, through its intervention in [...] an already structured field of knowledge'.[48] The already existing field of knowledge is the collection of other signifiers that make up the Symbolic order, represented in these diagrams as S^2. S^2 is the other to which S^1 is directed, it is the remainder of signifiers that organize around the master signifier to form knowledge. S^2 can be said to pre-exist the intervention of S^1 by virtue of the master signifier still being a signifier, it is thus part of this same series of signifiers before the intervention that privileges it over the other signifiers. This fact also eliminates any essential link between the signifier that performs the function of S^1 and the function itself: any signifier could, potentially, perform this ordering function. S^2 is, then, the order of knowledge put into operation by S^1, and the master signifier is what defines [S^2's] readability.[49] The neatness of this relation is troubled by the other two parts of the discourse; *a* in Lacan's schema comes in to stand for a surplus created during this production of knowledge, this is the surplus created by the inability for the relation between S^1 and S^2 to completely correspond with its aim. The aim of S^1, Lacan argues, 'is to represent the subject for another signifier'.[50] The subject is the $ located in the bottom left of the master's discourse in the place of truth. The subject is barred because of the split that language inaugurates in the subject: the signifier is inadequate to completely convey the totality of the subject's being. This process of representation fails because 'the subject it represents is not univocal. It is represented, undoubtedly, but also it is not represented. At this level, something remains hidden in relation to this very same signifier'.[51] What remains hidden is the part of the subject that the signifier cannot represent, and this failure is what produces the surplus. The production of *a*, an excess of enjoyment (*plus-de-jouir*), stands as a proof that the relation between S^1 and S^2 is not fixed or essential and that desire on the part of the subject is at play within the production of knowledge.[52] The discourse of the master in this sense is a failure: mastery can never be achieved because the subject can never be fully commensurate with her linguistic representation.

This failure of the master's command is supplemented by another structure of discourse that Lacan terms the discourse of the university and attributes the following graph to designate its structure:

$$\frac{\mathbf{S^2}}{\mathbf{S^1}} \rightarrow \frac{\boldsymbol{a}}{\mathbf{\$}}$$

Here in the position of agent is S^2, signifying knowledge. The other in this matrix upon which knowledge acts is *a*, surplus enjoyment, that is, all that remains outside the purview of S^2. Everything is subject to knowledge in the university discourse, and concomitantly, there is nothing that cannot be known. Lacan glosses the relation between S2 and *a* as such: 'It is impossible not to obey the commandment there in the place of what is the truth of science, "Continue. March on. Keep on knowing more and more"'.[53] The discourse of the university is then, in this respect, totalitarian, in that it demands full subjection of the totality of phenomena to reason/the signifier. The product of this relation is the subject, $. The subject produced is one amenable to the form of knowledge designated by S^2. Up to this point, knowledge would seem to function as a neutral category and the subject produced would be one perpetually more knowledgeable, a rational actor who would be able to make decisions based on the knowledge that is produced, that is, the form of subject described by utilitarianism. However, what complicates this process is the S^1 positioned at the bottom left of the matrix. The master signifier is at play in the university discourse, driving the entire process of knowledge production. As such, Lacan argues that 'the university has an extremely precise function, in effect, one that at every moment is related to the state we are in with respect to the master's discourse namely, its elucidation'.[54] What is enunciated in the university discourse is not objective truth but one 'related to the state we are in', meaning that knowledge conforms to a pre-existent demand, the master's discourse. The use of the term state also highlights an unacknowledged political aspect to the production of knowledge: knowledge is always politicized.[55] To build on my previous assertion that knowledge and power are not always imminent in each other, it is the university discourse that produces the link between power and knowledge. Within this structure of discourse, being as it is directed by a nonsensical demand, this link cannot be undone. As such, any critique of the university discourse obeys the master's demand to know more and thus maintains the power structure being critiqued.

The presence of an incoherent master as the source of the university discourse has an effect both on the form of knowledge being enunciated and the type of subject it produces. The form of knowledge produced is not knowledge of a truth outside of language. It is knowledge amenable to the originary demand of the master. Bruce Fink distinguishes the type of knowledge operative in the university discourse:

> We can imagine it not as the kind of thought that tries to come to grips with the real, to maintain the difficulties posed by apparent logical and/or physical contradictions but rather as a kind of encyclopaedic endeavour to exhaust a field.[56]

Two aspects of the university discourse become apparent from Fink's distinction. First is necessity for the field of knowledge to already be in place. It is towards that field that this form of knowledge returns to reconfirm its place. Nothing new enters into this circuit, what is enunciated is a reconfirmation of what was already known, that is, a repetition of the master signifier. Another aspect that is apparent is the process would seem to be infinite. The 'endeavour to exhaust a field' acts as an incitement to discourse that can never be fulfilled because more can always be said and studied and the field itself can, theoretically, be expanded and divided into infinitely more parts. Thus, what causes the master's discourse to fail, the disjunction between the subject's desire and the signifier, is also what allows the discourse of the university to continue indefinitely: the university thus translates the master's demand into law.[57]

The subject produced during this process is also linked to the master's presence. Whereas in the discourse of the master, the split subject taints the master's discourse with the presence of desire; in the university discourse, it is desire itself that is named by the signifier and the subject produced is one entirely amenable to the master's demand. The presence of the master's demand is what changes the subject from a rational actor capable of independent actions based upon objective realities, the utilitarian subject, into a docile body who is incited to discourse, to repeat the master's demand. In this way, the university completes the ambition of the master's discourse by producing a subject capable of repeating the forms of knowledge that bind it to the originary demand of the master. The product of the university discourse is not truth or knowledge, but rather, knowledge and truth are the means by which subjects are bound to the master. The master signifier then comes to be the means through which the subject learns to enjoy. This enjoyment is made manifest for the subject by the repetition of the master signifier, the incitement to discourse previously noted. This performative aspect, the continued avowal of power and its forms of knowledge, constitutes the means by which the discourse of the university repeats itself and thus maintains the hegemony of the master.

Two of the masters whose discourses dominate the trial were, as previously mentioned T.S. Eliot and F.R. Leavis. Both were asked to contribute to the case as expert witnesses. Leavis refused. In a letter for *The Spectator* written after the judgement, he explained both his reticence to bear testimony and to himself being witnesses his own discourse being appropriated by the defence:

> I express here, of course, my conviction that the outcome of the trial cannot at best be seen as pure gain [...]. [A] real advance, in the sense represented by Lawrence, depends upon the existence of a body of genuinely enlightened opinion, ensuring that the nature of Lawrence's genius and achievement shall he widely understood, so that these may have their proper force. *Lady Chatterley's Lover*, then—it is important that this obvious enough truth should be recognised--is a bad novel. Moreover, to assert, as was done again and again during the trial, and made a major point in the final speech for the Defence, that without having read it one cannot truly appreciate Lawrence's. Other work, and so cannot have received what the great and salutary creative writer of our time has to give, is to betray and further an alarming misconception of his genius and what he actually achieved; it is to misrepresent this disastrously. For the experts did not mean by their testimony that *Lady Chatterley's Lover*, in giving us something that violates Lawrence's own essential canons as an artist, serves as a foil to his successful and great art, and in that way may be used as an 'aid to its critical appreciation'. The book should be current as an unquestioned literary classic- -this was essential to the case for the Defence.[58]

The fundamental reason for Leavis's refusal to testify on behalf of the defence was his refusal to accede to the importance, and, by extension, the literary merit of *Lady Chatterley's Lover.* For Leavis, the novel is a 'bad novel' that is emblematic of Lawrence's oeuvre as a whole. One of the defence's key arguments was that publishing the novel would allow readers to understand Lawrence fully for the first time. Here, Leavis's view directly contradicts their message. What seems to have most irked Leavis is the improper reading of Lawrence that he frames as a 'misconception of his genius', a 'misrepresent[ation]' and a 'betray[l]'. The expert witnesses have given false witness to the truth of the text and to Lawrence.

The majority of the witnesses who gave testimony and the defence council themselves had based their arguments on those in Leavis's criticism.[59] It is then not the misconception of Lawrence that so appals Leavis but rather the perceived misconception of his own discourse on display at the trial that Leavis finds so distasteful. The discourse of the master functioning in his absence is out of his control. The trial for Leavis would then be an encounter with his own impotency, his inability to control the dissemination and interpretation of his own enunciation. And as we can see from the success of the defence's argumentation, the fact that the argument functions more smoothly without him. This is the first instance in the trial of the (symbolic) death of the master facilitating the formation of a stable body of knowledge: the arbitrary nature of Leavis's claims to the truth of a text, grounded in citation of Lawrence, actually makes him a liability. Instead, Leavis is reduced to citation, the citation being much more malleable than the man himself. His absence allows for a consistent claim to the text's truth. If the master is to be present in the discourse of the university, it is only at a symbolic level, the subject who enunciated that discourse finds himself silenced.

T.S. Eliot's criticism proved to be much more problematic for the defence. As mentioned previously, Eliot had previously been heavily critical of Lawrence, so much so that *D.H. Lawrence Novelist*, upon which the defence and the expert witnesses based their testimony, can be seen as direct rebuttal of Eliot's statements on Lawrence. As such, Eliot was included in a list drawn up of 'hostile' critics of Lawrence who were deemed to be liable to be cited by the Prosecution for the purposes of disproving literary merit. This made the potential testimony of Eliot both dangerous and valuable to the defence. If they could persuade Eliot to renege on his previous claims, they could disrupt any potential use by the prosecution of Eliot as a claim to truth in regard to *Lady Chatterley*'s Obscenity. And, in doing so, usurp that authority for their own ends. The discourse of the master had value if it could be shown to have changed. But by virtue of its claim to mastery, the sovereignty of its claim to truth, the process of changing would signal an inconsistency in the master himself and by extension an inconsistency in the claim to truth or in the field of knowledge he institutes through his claim.

Eliot was asked by the prosecution to bear witness but refused, instead, after much deliberation, decided to bear witness for the defence. In a letter to Helen Gardener, Eliot detailed his motivations behind offering his testimony at the trial:

> My feeling about Lawrence remain ambiguous and my desire to give witness was really rather a protest against other books, such as *Lolita*, which struck me as really evil, which much more deserve censoring. The great pity is that the Crown chose Lawrence's book for prosecution. One knows what will happen: once a book has been under the charge of obscenity not even a jury can give absolution, and the book will be bought by thousands who are quite incapable of understanding what Lawrence was after.[60]

Eliot admits to a persistent ambiguity as regards his own critical judgement of Lawrence: in *After Strange Gods*, his stated position is hostile whilst in the witness proofs prepared for the trial, his position is one of admiration. Eliot confesses to a failure of his critical judgement in classifying Lawrence, an inability to categorize within literary and moral terms the essence of his texts. Knowing that the law demands a clear demarcation of the subject's position, this ambivalence makes testimony for the prosecution or defence impossible in the sense that Eliot's ambiguity positions him between these competing claims to the truth of Lawrence's text. Eliot, in contrast to Leavis, allows himself to bear what would seem to be false witness to this ambiguity by siding with the defence. The justification for this deception is a seemingly greater ethical problem and an apparently much more dangerous text: Vladimir Nabokov's *Lolita*. *Lolita*, unlike Lawrence's text, is 'really evil' and 'much more deserving of censoring'. Again, the problem for Eliot, as can be seen in many other of the defenders of *Lady Chatterley*, is not so much censorship itself but the erroneous reading of texts by those 'quite incapable of understanding' the serious and decent literary essence of Lawrence and the dangerous *jouissance* that books like *Lolita* embodied. The problem for Eliot, as it almost always is in his criticism, is that of improper or perverse reading, and by extension, the proper and improper enjoyment wrought by the text.

For the same reason, Eliot constituted a valuable witness for the defence, his testimony presented problems to the defence's narrative and strategy. Similarly to Leavis, Eliot too had to encounter an interpretation of himself in the domain of the other, quite contrary to his own convictions, and wished to correct them. His statements regarding Lawrence in *After Strange Gods* marked him out as hostile towards Lawrence and therefore could be used as potential evidence for the prosecution, as a counter-argument to positive criticism of Lawrence, as well as damaging the defence's strategy of a united front as regards the field of literary criticism's appreciation of Lawrence: if somebody as influential as Eliot disagreed with the other critic's assessment of Lawrence, then in no way could the text be said to be said to have objective literary merit. As such, Eliot and the defence had to form an argument that both dealt with the potentially damning portions of Eliot's criticism of Lawrence whilst also distancing themselves from that position. A series of witness proofs were drawn up for his statement in court. It is to those that I now wish to turn.

As with the majority of expert witnesses called by the defence Eliot's testimony begins with a long series of accolades and achievements that legitimize his position as an expert in his field. With many of the witnesses, these declarations of expertise mobilized disciplinary discourses that the defence used in order to claim the literary merit, and thus, the disciplinary value of Lawrence's text. The discourse of nation is repeated numerous times in these introductions in numerous forms: place of birth, educational and religious institutions as well as, where possible, military experience, specifically focused on duties during the Second World War. The tactic appears to be not only the garnering of nationalistic sympathy from the jurors but also to implicate the discourse of literary criticism within the discourse of nationalism much like Leavis's attempts with Lawrence's texts. These witnesses thus represent England and its assumed, but crucially unspoken, values as much as they do literary criticism. Lawrence, by extension, can also be said to come to be representative of these values, his writing is then representative of English literature but also, crucially, a remedy for English society. His exclusion would do irreparable harm. The emphasis on nation and the military in these opening statements thus has a key pharmacological function, modifying the foreign threatening elements of Lawrence's text by signifying both its Englishness and its vital potential to eliminate any potential threats to English society.

But therein lies the fundamental ambiguity of Eliot and his place with the domain of English literature: his status as a major poet and theorist of English literature and his established presence in English literary culture contrasts with his status as a foreigner. Eliot's American heritage marks him as an outsider, a foreign body that potentially pollutes the emphasis on the Englishness of the witnesses so carefully managed by the defence. Care is taken in the list of qualifications to anglicize Eliot as much as possible. His naturalization as a British subject in 1927 is the first detailed in his introduction. Numerous references to British universities are mentioned where possible. However, the cosmopolitan make-up of Eliot's education is still very much evident. These numerous degrees from Europe and America are useful in that they go some way to justifying Eliot's status as a master in that confer upon him a cross-cultural and thus conceivably objective status as a master of his field. However, this appeal to the outside for confirmation of the legitimacy and autonomy of English literature troubles the attempts to cordon off the subject and the texts of Lawrence within a purely English context. The performance of mastery heightens Eliot's value as a witness whilst simultaneously devaluing the defence's strategy and claim to truth. Eliot's position as both a Churchwarder and Vice President of the Church Union reaffirms his Englishness by attaching him to the Church of England and also locates himself and his work within the Christian morality in which the defence also wished to place Lawrence and his texts. His position as President of the London Library and director of Faber and Faber, based in London, also helps to domesticate his foreignness. Thus, Eliot's testimony, from the introduction, initiates a pharmacology: both his foreignness and his past hostility constitute potentially toxic elements which need to be mitigated and filtered in order for his testimony to be beneficial for the defence's purpose.

Similar to the introductory statements, the main body of the statement begins by directly confronting one of the major sources of anxiety in relation to Eliot's history, his criticism of Lawrence in *After Strange Gods*. The criticism therein is immediately mitigated by the admission that due to another lecture course being written at the same time, Eliot could not 'give enough time to either book as [he] would have liked'. Thus begins a series of attempts to distance Eliot's current position from those found in *After Strange Gods*, which in another sense constitutes a distinction between the text that appears under his name and the speaking subject who would give testimony in 1960. To begin in this manner, an admission that the masterly pronouncements of that text were, in truth, unfinished or not fit for publication, is an ambiguous strategy: in the first instance, it achieves the goal of distancing the truth claims made in *After Strange Gods* from the opposing truth claims being constructed by the defence. But in the process of this distancing or adulteration, the position of Eliot as master, a subject with access to truth, is likewise undercut. An attempt is made to reassert mastery in response to this loss of sovereignty over the field by the admission that Eliot himself recognized his own error as ceased publication of the lectures. The emphasis placed in the witness proof on the small amounts of copies produced of *After Strange Gods*, 4,500 in total, serves to both display Eliot's power over the dissemination of his texts and dissuade any anxieties about that dissemination; the risk of the text reaching the wrong reader is presented as unlikely and Eliot has done all in his power to mitigate that risk. In all of this positioning what is of key importance is the anxiety provoked by the free flow of the signifier absent of the agency of a subject, the signifier divorced from life. Eliot's testimony represents a struggle between the master and his enunciation for sovereignty over meaning. The excess produced in the discourse of the master, the excess of meaning in his enunciation that signals his impotence is itself the target of Eliot's statement: it is the attempted refusal of the master to die.

Eliot makes the case that Lawrence's importance, and thus literary merit, is implied in the act of criticism itself by stating that he would 'not have wasted [his] time lecturing upon him and comparing him to James Joyce and others if I had not considered him a most important writer of English and of most influence on English Literature'. Here, the justification of Lawrence's merit is based upon Eliot's perceived authority upon the field of literary criticism. 'Influence' is an ambiguous term that can be positive or negative depending on how it is perceived as we can see in the numerous interpretations of the corrupting influence of texts. Here, it is the value of Eliot as master that confers a positive connotation to the word influence. The value of Eliot's enunciation is also what determines the value of both Joyce and Lawrence. Eliot's reading and subsequent enunciation of a truth claim about them, even if that claim is negative, gives these authors their literary merit. However, it is this very act of criticism that Eliot is seeking to disavow; thus, the value of Eliot's criticism has also come into question. A reversal is engendered, whereby the value of Eliot's claim to mastery is now dependent upon the perceived value of Lawrence's text; accordingly, Eliot must seek to modify his own claims to better fit this narrative.

Thus, begins a series of battles between the master and his unruly citations. Eliot's witness proof morphs into a piece of Lawrence criticism 'on the literary merit of *Lady Chatterley's Lover*'. Following each citation, he comments on, qualifies, 'disown[s]' and disavows the positions enunciated in the citation in an attempt to both justify his own position as legitimate expert and in order to justify Lawrence's text in the terms by which the defence's case is figured.

Eliot outlines the major forms of heresy he previously detected in Lawrence's work. Key to his critique is the detection of a 'strain of morbidity in [Lawrence's] work' and in particular a 'distinct sexual morbidity'. This analysis, the presence of disease and death as the essence of Lawrence's texts, directly contravenes the defence's framing of the text as palliative, the essentially healthy and normative aspect of Lawrence's writing. To link this presence of death in the text to sexuality further contradicts the narrative framing of sexuality and Lawrence's representation of it. Lawrence's intense investment in the sexual act and the sex scenes of *Lady Chatterley's Lover* were to be depicted as examples of healthy relations towards bodies and the sexes: sex, in this sense, comes to figure a denial of death. But Eliot detects in Lawrence the presence of death underwriting his stated investment in life, speculating in the proof that he 'might have progressed beyond from his early belief in Life to a belief in Death'.

This ambivalent aspect of Lawrence, the constant oscillations between life and death, creativity and destruction, desire and disgust, have been shown to be at work in *The Rainbow* in the first chapter of this thesis and the detection of which were a major deciding factor towards its categorization as obscene. In that chapter, Lawrence's texts were brought into dialogue with the psychoanalytic concept of the death drive that, in Sabina Spielrein's words, marks 'the destructive component of the sexual instinct'.[61] For Spielrein, and later Freud, sex comes to represent a crucial problem in that the creative act of sexuality, a force that connects the subject and the other, cannot be separated from a destructive and solitary form of enjoyment, the drive. Eliot's diagnosis differs from the psychoanalytic insight in that it informs a specific critique of Lawrence's texts as pathological exceptions from the proper or orthodox mode of literature. The presence of death in these texts is not itself a norm but evidence of Lawrence's 'monstrosity'. This presence of the drive is also present in Lawrence's apparent 'insensibility to ordinary morality', the existence of his characters and by extension the texts themselves outside the orthodox Christian morality not only prevents incorporation within the tradition of English literature but also 'baffles' Eliot, potentially disrupting the body of knowledge that his critical writing labours to maintain.

The connection between Lawrence's perceived sickness and his representation of sexuality is given a further dimension in Eliot's analysis of the class and gender dynamics in *Lady Chatterley*, *The Virgin and the Gypsy* and *The Plumed Serpent*. In *After Strange Gods*, Eliot argues that Lawrence's working-class origin and his resentment towards the middle classes produces in his work 'the social obsession which makes (Lawrence's) well-born – or almost well-born – ladies offer themselves to – or make use of – plebeians', and that this impulse to engage in the improper mixing of classes 'springs from the same morbidity which make other of his female characters bestow their favours on savages'.[62] Here, the sexual relations between working-class men and women of the upper classes is symptomatic of a larger sickness at play in Lawrence's work: Eliot detects a certain desire in Lawrence to humiliate these women through sexual relations with these men in order to destroy their socially instituted superiority, these relations thus become a form of revenge upon these women and their class in general. Ultimately, the source of this sickness is located in the author himself when Eliot declares: 'The author of this book seems to me to have been a very sick man indeed'.[63] And Lawrence's sickness ran the risk of contagion to his readers, as Eliot goes on to argue:

'I fear that Lawrence's work may appeal, not to those who are well and able to discriminate, but to the sick and debile and confused; and will appeal not to what remains of health in them, but to their sickness'.[64] This sickness, this lack of social propriety and excess of sexual enjoyment at work in the text, that causes Eliot such anxiety is thus given a source, Lawrence himself and his texts thus function as vectors for the spread of this sickness to the multitude of his readers. In this sense, Eliot's criticism functions as a form of literary pathology, hunting for symptoms of sickness and tracing their sources and causes. To declare the source of this illness as the author himself succeeds in immunizing literature and its readers from this disruptive foreign body.

The strategy of immunization is, according to Roberto Esposito, key to understanding how biopolitics functions in such a way as to mobilize 'all of knowledge and power's dispositifs [to create a] protective containment in the face of a vital power that is led to expand without limits'.[65] It is this vital power that ceases to stop growing that I have variously referred to in this chapter as *bios* or the drive. Here, in Esposito, this unruly force constitutes a threat to communal life:

> immunitas is revealed as the negative or lacking form of communitas. If communitas is that relation, which in binding its members to an obligation of reciprocal donation, jeopardizes individual identity, immunitas is the condition of dispensation from such an obligation and therefore the defense against the expropriating features of communitas. [...] One can say that generally immunitas, to the degree it protects the one who bears it from risky contact with those who lack it, restores its own borders that were jeopardized by the common.[66]

Immunitas is thus a component of *communitas*, the means by which it protects itself from contact and infection from foreign bodies, it creates and protects borders. But much like in Agamben's dynamic between the sovereign and *homo sacer*, in a sense *immunitas* comes to name both the sovereign who decides the exception and the exception itself: both the sovereign and the foreign body are outside the *communitas* instituting a dimension of the undecidable wherein that very body whose individuality is represented in the figure of the sovereign and protected by borders, becomes aware of its own impossibility and corruption from without and within.

> What is immunized [...] is the same community in a form that both preserves and negates it, or better, preserves it through the negation of its original horizon of sense. From this point of view, one might say that more than the defensive apparatus superimposed on the community, immunization is its internal mechanism: the fold that in some way separates community from itself, sheltering it from an unbearable excess.[67]

This unbearable excess would be precisely that aspect of the sexual, the life creating force, that contains within the deathly dimension of the drive. In any attempt to delineate the borders between outside and inside, subject and other, nation and foreigner, an 'unbearable excess' emerges from within those borders. This excess is also a recognition of the lack of the defining features of *communitas* that distinguish it from the foreign body.

Commenting on Esposito's work, Eric Santner argues that in

> this conception of an "immunological dialectic" whereby shelter becomes its own kind of life-threatening exposure, immunity becomes autoimmunity, self-preservation becomes a mode of mortification, life drive becomes a kind of death drive, [...] something falls through the cracks of the dialectic and keeps returning to its place to initiate the whole process again, indeed to endow it with the aspect of a repetition compulsion.[68]

The impossibility of these borders' maintenance engenders a form of paranoia in which the foreign body is perpetually located and abjected from the communitas. This compulsion to repeat signals the work of the drive at the very heart of the attempt to preserve and continue life: sickness underwriting health.

Something akin to this dynamic emerges in Eliot's battle with his citations. In his efforts to maintain the boundaries between orthodox and heretical writing Eliot, functioning as sovereign, diagnoses within Lawrence's texts a certain threat to *communitas*, the shared experiences he defines as a 'living tradition'. Lawrence's texts threaten such life with spiritual illness. The immunological manoeuvre is thus to locate that illness with Lawrence the subject. As I have hitherto mentioned, the author as the location of the source of ultimate meaning for a text functions as a supplement for a perceived unbearable non-presence at the core of the signifier. This sickness that Eliot locates in Lawrence, I wish to argue, is an effect of signification apparent in his texts but by no means unique to them.

In his witness proof, Eliot declares that this decision was one he regretted and considered 'much too violent'. In his subsequent revision of this decision, a reversal takes place in which the contagion once located in Lawrence is now evident in the *communitas:* 'It is my opinion now that it may be our society which is morbid and sick in its attitude to sex rather than Lawrence'. The morbidity previously diagnosed in *Lady Chatterley* is now recognized in society, with the novel now transformed into a form of medicine from which 'There are certainly moral lessons to be learned'. The reversal in the sovereign decision engenders a reversal in the location of the sickness, and the excess cannot be fully eliminated but rather moves from one zone to its opposite. Again, it is sex that functions as the locus for the emergence of this sickness: in both of Eliot's diagnoses, someone, somewhere is doing sex wrong, is enjoying the wrong way.

Finally, a third location of sickness is located by Eliot: the master himself. In order to explain the reason behind his violent decisions, Eliot recalls his personal experiences at the time of the lectures and their subsequent publication and, in doing so, admits to the presence of desire, and thus inconsistency, functioning at the level of the master's discourse:

> I should mention that there were events in my private life which I can see in retrospect affected my critical judgement and made me more sweeping and violent in my assertions than I now feel.
>
> One of those particularly unhappy periods was about 1929–1934 and during this period when I lectured about Lawrence and prepared AFTER STRANGE GODS for publication in 1933, I should have realised that I as well as he, should have described as "a sick soul".

In disclosing these facts, Eliot collapses the distinction between the inner private life of the subject and the public discourse of the master, admitting that the desires and circumstances of the former determine the judgements contained in the latter. The decisions of the master that claim impartiality are thus dependent upon a desiring subject and therefore cannot claim to be impartial. The period of time Eliot stated in his proof corresponds to a period of conflict his first wife Vivienne Haigh-Wood Eliot which would result in them separating in 1933 and ending in her being committed to an asylum. By bringing in this period as a potential reason for his judgement, Eliot alludes to a sexual influence behind his judgement thus implicating sexuality itself as sustaining the master's discourse. Additionally, this sexual aspect is not healthy or beneficial and results in 'sweeping and violent [...] assertions'. The sexual aspect underwriting the master's discourse harms Eliot's position as impartial master, and that this sexual aspect is defined by him as destructive runs contrary to the defence's framing of sexuality as a positive and healthy aspect of life.

It is also this presence of the sexual that results in a complete reversal in the location of the sickness that Eliot located in Lawrence originally. From immunizing the society from the destructive *jouissance* of Lawrence's text by locating that *jouissance* in Lawrence, the sickness then moves into the community itself with Lawrence's text acting as a potential cure. Finally, that sickness comes to be located in Eliot himself as he comes to identify with that destructive *jouissance* that he had attempted to renounce in the abjection of Lawrence from the tradition. Eliot's desire for the absolution of *Lady Chatterley's Lover* can perhaps then be reformulated as desire for the personal absolution of his 'sick soul' from this unbearable *jouissance*. The elusive excess which his criticism continually renounced in other texts is, upon confrontation with his own citation, found in himself. The proof is then a form of confession from the master reluctantly acknowledging his own failure.

What provides the basis for this disruption of the categories of life and death, health and sickness, and self and other is presence of the sexual, or, rather, the renunciation of the disruptive aspect of sexuality. Eliot's confrontation with the relation between sexuality, the signifier and truth effects a number of disruptions and reversals at odds with the defence's presentation of a repressed society in need of an injection of healthy sexuality. It is not the sickness of society or the need for intervention that Eliot's proof disagrees with but rather the rigour of his auto-criticism betrays the inconsistencies inherent within sexuality itself. The discourse of the master cannot curtail this antagonistic element of sexuality: the ability to manage this unruly object will be a key aspect to the discourse of the university and the use of psychiatric discourses in the trial proper.

The university discourse shares with obscenity law the function of regulating and policing desire. Enjoyment in the form of the *object a* in the master's discourse indicates the failure of the master's speech because his discourse is always implicated in structures of desire that exceed the signifier's ability to represent them. In the university discourse, the enjoyment that signalled the failure of the master now becomes the object that is acted upon, managed, codified and domesticated by the signifier. It is this process that Foucault in *The History of Sexuality* names '*Scientia Sexualis*'.[69] According to Foucault, the 19th and 20th centuries bore witness to an ever-increasing 'policing of sex' whose main aim was not repression or taboo but rather 'regulating sex through useful and public discourses'.[70] Sex is subjected to knowledge and is thus rendered both useful and public. Sex becomes part of *bios*, and the subject's relation to it becomes the means by which they can be judged as productive members of society or excluded for having an unhealthy relationship to sex. The subject must perform her sex for others, and this performance is enjoyable. What is occurring here is a neutralization of desire in its complexity to a very narrow definition of sexuality. *Jouissance*, properly policed, becomes sexuality. Foucault, in an essay discussing sexuality in the work of Georges Bataille, characterizes this process as a violent effect of discourse:

> What characterizes modern sexuality [...] is not its having found the language of its logic or of its natural process, but rather, through the violence done by such languages, its having been "denatured"-cast into an empty

> zone where it achieves whatever meagre form is bestowed upon it by the establishment of its limits. Sexuality points to nothing beyond itself.[71]

As with Lacan's definition of the university discourse, sexuality in Foucault's argument is an object of knowledge that 'points to nothing beyond itself'. The naturalness and 'logic' that discourse ascribes to its object of study is typified by Foucault as a form of violence that masks the agency of the signifier in producing that very logic: sexuality is not a truth latent in each subject awaiting discovery and definition, but it is a product of signification. This process has as its ultimate aim 'the establishment of limits'. That limit appears to be the subject itself, or rather the subject that emerges as the product of the university discourse: if sexuality points to nothing but itself and the truth of the subject resides in her sexuality, then the aim of the discourses of sexuality that Foucault describes is the production of individualized subjects, themselves 'denatured'. In a sense, these sexual subjects are also sexless: their sexuality cannot move beyond the narrow scope of permissible sexual practices that confirm their status as a subject.

This notion of sex as an object of knowledge contrasts with the psychoanalytic understanding of sex as a disruptive force, signalling the impossibility of those very fields of knowledge that a *Scientia Sexualis* attempts to capture it within. Zupančič argues that:

> in psychoanalysis sex is above all a concept that formulates a persisting contradiction of reality. [...] [T]his contradiction cannot be circumscribed or reduced to a secondary level (as a contradiction between already well-established entities/beings), but is—as a contradiction—involved in the very structuring of these entities, in their very being. In this precise sense, sex is of ontological relevance: not as an ultimate reality, but as an inherent twist, or stumbling block, of reality.[72]

Sex, in this understanding, cannot be reduced to an object of study among others, that is, reduced to sense, tamed by language. Sex is immanent in reality in so far as it is also, to borrow Copjec's phrase, 'the stumbling block of sense'[73]: if sexuality is immanent, the very way we attempt to understand the world, then any attempt to circumscribe it within a body of knowledge, within language, must either fail or, as Foucault suggests, necessarily denature the sexual so as to make it amenable to knowledge, thus the emphasis within *Scientia Sexualis* upon sexual practices as an observable and quantifiable manifestation of sex. A fantasy emerges here of a desexualized science capable of, like the master's discourse, objective truths, but unlike the master, these truths are not undermined by the presence of sexuality because sex itself is neutralized as another form of knowledge.

Zupančič goes on to state what psychoanalysis shares with modern science but also where it differs:

> Psychoanalysis is *both* coextensive with this desexualisation of reality, in the sense of breaking with ontology and science as a sexual technique or sexual combinatory, *and* absolutely uncompromising when it comes to the sexual as the irreducible *Real* (not substance).[74]

It is then psychoanalysis's refusal to conceive of sex as a substance that can be isolated or located in specific practices and techniques that differentiates it from *Scientia Sexualis*. With this in mind, the accusation that psychoanalysis also constitutes a form of *Scientia Sexualis* that incites a confession from the analysand in order to locate their truth in their sexual practices falters because, in psychoanalysis, sex cannot function as the locus of truth for the subject but rather the impossibility of locating any form of truth within the subject herself.[75] If a truth claim can be made by psychoanalysis about the subject, it can only be about the subject's specific relation to their lack of truth.

What allows this distinction to emerge is the specific relation to language taken by the university discourse and psychoanalysis. By having knowledge play the role of agent in the interrogation of desire, the status of knowledge as language and therefore subject to the vicissitudes of desire must be repressed. Language in the university discourse is conceived as the means through which the communication of information occurs free of the stain of desire which has been segregated into an object of knowledge. In this schema, any lack or excess does not intimate a constitutive deadlock; instead, these interruptions and contradictions initiate the incitement for further discourse. The university discourse's operative fantasy is the entirety of being under the control of the signifier: it imagines the complete eradication of the other and the dictatorship of the rational self. Psychoanalysis takes a very different approach to language. The excesses and gaps that appear in discourse, the disruptions of symbolic reality are interpreted as symptoms of a gap operative in the function of speech. Lacan elucidates on this gap by arguing that:

> discourse begins from the fact that there is a gap here.[...] But, after all, nothing prevents us from saying that it is because discourse begins that the gap is produced. It is a matter of complete indifference towards the result. What is certain is that discourse is implied in the gap.[76]

As to whether the gap pre-exists discourse or is in fact produced by discourse is of little consequence for Lacan. The importance lies in inferring that this undecidability emerges in the event of discourse's failure, this failure of discourse is indicative of a gap. And it is in relation to this gap that sex emerges as a compensatory force. Zupančič, following on from Lacan, argues that sex 'emerges only from, and at the place of, this lack, and attempts to deal with it. [I]t is [...] the messy sewing up of this gap'.[77] Sex can then be understood as the force that attempts to suture the gap between the subject and the other that discourse's failure announces: sex is an attempt to save the One. But, in this attempt, to save the One, a surplus of enjoyment emerges in the subject's discourse, the *object a*. This disruptive element of sexuality is the major difference between *Scientia Sexualis* and psychoanalysis. *Scientia Sexualis* is an attempt to sort out the mess and use sex as a locus of truth, thereby suturing the gap in discourse: it is invested in the fantasy of the One and labours to maintain it. Psychoanalysis in comparison sees in sexuality that 'what splits into two is the very nonexistence of the one'.[78] Psychoanalysis, in comparison to the university discourse, does not attempt to bridge this gap but instead remains attentive to this gap and to the mess that compensates for it. For both, sexuality functions as a problem but where they differ is that, for psychoanalysis, '[s]exuality is the paradigm of research and exploration, not in the sense of the reduction to the last instance but, on the contrary, because it brutally introduces us to the lack of the last instance'.[79]

In this way, we can trace an overlap between the policing of desires that Foucault attributes to biopolitics and the discourse of the university described by Lacan. The work of reparation enacted by *Scientia Sexualis* upon sex, its neutralization and utilization, goes towards the creation of a subject whose truth is located in their desire and sexual practices. The desire of the subject then becomes a quantifiable measurement of the subject. This helps with the management of populations in a way that the law previously could not maintain: the subject now finds that her desire is her responsibility; it is her duty to confess her desire in acts that are appropriate to her true self. It is no longer the law's function to police proper forms of enjoyment, but rather it is the subject's duty to be true to herself in all that she consumes, practices and enjoys.

The absence of a locus of truth in which to ground the subject's truth and the disruptive aspect of sexuality are the two major points in which psychoanalysis deviates from modern science and are also the two aspects of sexuality that the defence's use of psychiatric expert witnesses attempts to elide. I wish to argue that the trial stages a transition of the duty of policing the subject's enjoyment of literary texts from the state and legislature, discourses of the master, onto the literary critic and the discourse of the university.

If, as Sean Matthews argues, the trial 'consistently blurred the distinction between court and classroom', and this is because the two discourses not only share similar reading practices that aim at discerning a true judgement of the facts but also share a similar aim: the codification of knowledge and the management of enjoyment.[80] The shared concerns of both discourses are made apparent by two significant questions that the trial provokes: what is good writing? What is good sex? The trial links these two concerns around the notion of public good. The defence's tactic in this case was to fully exploit this aspect of the new legislation. Their tactic was to mobilize as many experts in as many fields as possible to show a united front as regards the effect of Lawrence's text: *Lady Chatterley* was good for you because it represented sexuality in a healthy way that would benefit both the subject reading the text and English culture at large. Lawrence according to this reading was an agent of sexual liberation, releasing the subject from repression. Sexuality would have to be figured by the defence as a form of civic enjoyment needing expression, the health of the nation would depend upon it. As such, the defence would have to navigate the class and gender anxieties that the previous legislation had enshrined. Whereas the previous legislation had figured working class and female sexuality as a threat to the national body, in this reading, these subjects are now invited to enjoy *for* the nation, providing that it was the right kind of enjoyment based upon the right kind of reading. This new framing of the reader was in keeping with the structure of the university discourse as described by Lacan and the biopolitics of Foucault: the defence posited a universal subject defined by their sexuality for whom repression of their sexuality posed a threat to themselves and society at large.

As demonstrated in previous chapters, literature has often been accused of corrupting the subject by introducing an improper enjoyment. This enjoyment was framed in all cases as potentially harmful to the social link between subjects. In most of these cases, this improper form of enjoyment was felt to be sexual in some way, and this form of sexuality posed a threat to normative sexual relations, what I have previously referred to, drawing on Lacanian psychoanalysis, as the sexual relation: in this sense, the improper enjoyment introduced by the literary text in the previous trials not only threatened the sexual relation but also in the trials themselves bore witness to the non-existence of the sexual relation itself. But in the *Lady Chatterley* trial, the defence attempts to reverse this dynamic by claiming that the form of enjoyment produced by *Lady Chatterley's Lover* was socially beneficial and the attempts to censor the text were in fact detrimental to the nation's health. In order to make this argument, the defence focused specifically on the sexual aspect on Lawrence's texts claiming that these aspects of the text did not signify perversity but rather honesty and bravery in the face of repressive forces both social and psychic.

In targeting sexual repression as the true enemy to the nation's health, the defence mobilized the discourse of psychiatry and psychoanalysis. But in order to argue that the literary text had the ability to lift repression from the subject thus allowing them to be liberated and fully enjoy, the defence had to construct an understanding of repression that allowed such a dynamic. Therefore, the psychiatric professionals called forth to be witnesses were specially chosen in order to substantiate this claim. It is then, as in the case of Eliot, instructive to examine the potential witnesses who were not called to testify just as much as those that were in order to better understand how the defence's claim to truth was produced: in other words, it can help us understand what has to be repressed in order to claim to understand repression.

In a letter to Ronald Hargreaves, Professor of Psychiatry at the University of Leeds, the defence clearly state their formulation of the relation between repression and the literary text:

> In this case there are psychiatric questions upon which you would clearly be an expert. I am advised by several psychiatrists that neurotics suffering

> from sexual obsessions have generally, in not invariably, been troubled by the suppression of guilty feelings when knowledge of sex has been obtained furtively and in connection with the "dirty" use of four letter words and so on.
>
> These experts consider that as regards such people, "Lady Chatterley's Lover" would be likely to do good, as bringing out into the open in a "clean" context, the matters which remain troublesome only when they are thought about furtively.

First, it is clear that the defence already have their conception of the role of repression in place and that Hargreaves is not so much being asked his opinion but rather if his understanding of repression fits in with this preconceived notion, garnered from other experts: his value as a potential witness stems not his own understanding of repression but his use value in repeating the defence's tactical definition. As regards that definition, sexuality itself is not being figured as the dirty content but the process by which the knowledge is kept secret bestows upon it its corrupted 'furtive' character. It follows that the clean is not a space absent of sexuality; instead, it is a place absent of repression where the truth of sexuality can be perceived and understood in a mature and healthy manner. The process of repression is the corrupting element, obscuring sexuality and forcing any confrontation with it to be done in secret. The function of the literary text then is to enact this process of purification by removing repression and transforming the dirty furtive secret of sex into clean, open and public knowledge. This conception of repression mirrors the Enlightenment conception of knowledge that conceives of reason penetrating the darkness of ignorance: the discourse of the university is thus operative in the defence's conception of repression as a corrupting force that requires combatting in the name of the public good.

Implicit within this framework is also a relation to literature and the signifier in general. The four-letter words function here as both catalysts and symptoms of a repressed knowledge about sexuality. The subject who understands sexuality in relation to these signifiers is classified as neurotic. By contrast, the literary text functions as a means to the appearance of the truth into the open thus alleviating the subject of their 'troublesome' neurosis. The subject's relation to sex can either be inauthentic or authentic, true or false. The pharmacological dimension becomes apparent in this differentiation between the dirty words of the working classes and the clean institution of literature: there are bad signifiers and good signifiers and the means by which we can distinguish them is by their relation to truth. The signifier's status as *pharmakon* is thus elided by the introduction of truth as a supplement. A tension emerges here, however. In order to function as a form of truth, the text's status as fiction must also be repressed. Added to this, if obscene words signal a neurotic relation to sexuality, then Lawrence's use of those words as a palliative to sexual repression seems destined to fail this tension also finds itself unaddressed in the defence's formulation of sexual repression.

The defence's position in regard to literature and sexual repression seems to be taken from Lawrence's text itself. In a passage from the final edition, the narrator discusses the potentially emancipatory effects of the novel:

> [T]he novel, properly handled [,][...] can inform and lead into new places the flow of our sympathetic consciousness, and it can lead our sympathy away in recoil from things gone dead. Therefore, the novel, properly handled, can reveal the most secret places of life: for it is in the *passional* secret places of life, above all, that the tide of sensitive awareness needs to ebb and flow, cleansing and freshening.[81]

The literary text can function here as a catalyst for purification, moving the reader away from death and into a more intimate relation with life's secret places, those previously hidden. This dynamic is framed in terms of a moral necessity, the passional or sexual forces require emancipation, and it is the proper place of the novelist to enact this movement away from death towards life. It could then be argued that the defence's rhetoric in defence of *Lady Chatterley* is but a textual echo of the text itself. But what this reading would miss out is the necessary repressions of the text itself that are required. The very next paragraph in the text lays out a double to the properly handled novel, the novel of improper and deathly enjoyment:

> But the novel, like gossip, can also excite spurious sympathies and recoils, mechanical and deadening to the psyche. The novel can glorify the most corrupt feelings, so long as they are *conventionally* 'pure'. Then the novel, like gossip, becomes at last vicious, and, like gossip, all the more vicious because it is always ostensibly on the side of the angels.[82]

This other novel excites 'spurious sympathies', enjoyment in non-truth, the mechanical and ultimately enjoyment in death. This deathly aspect of literature is all the more 'vicious' due to its ability to camouflage itself in convention, to pass as pure whilst 'glorify[ing] the most corrupt feelings'. What marks out this improper novel is its ability to equivocate, that is its ability to bear witness to the ambiguity of the signifier. This fundamental ambiguity of the signifier marks a profound disruption in the distinction between the good novel on the side of life and the improper, deathly novel. For if the novel is constructed of signifiers, and signifiers can appear goodly only to be deathly, then how can the reader ever know whether what they are reading is on the side of life or death: what exactly are they enjoying? It is precisely this undecidable aspect of the *pharmakon* that the process of pharmacology represses and, in the case of the *Lady Chatterley* trial, is the aspect of literature that is elided in their use of the concept of repression.

Repression for the defence was conceived as a product of societal pressures, or more precisely, society's ignorance, but the locus of repression was the subject herself: one either has a repressed relation to one's own sex or an enlightened relation but either way it belongs to the subject. The subject's relationship to the signifier is symptomatic of her relation to her own sexual truth. Implicit within this dynamic is the belief that the antagonistic element located in the sexual is a product of its repression rather than sex being the source of that conflict itself. As discussed above, where psychoanalysis differs from the defence's form of repression, wherein the subject is wholly responsible for their relationship to sexuality, it conceives of repression as constitutive of both the subject and the signifying order itself. In his essay 'Repression', Freud theorizes what he terms 'primal repression':

> We have reason to assume that there is a primal repression, a first phase of repression, which consists in the psychical (ideational) representative of the instinct being denied entrance into the conscious. With this fixation is established; the representative in question persists unaltered from then onwards and the instinct remains attached to it.[83]

What is denied access to the conscious is the representative an instinct or, in another register, a signifier that would complete the circuit of the drive: this drive becomes fixed in a repetitive motion unable to find closure except in repeating itself. Primal repression can then be understood not as an event in the subject's life that can be reversed, but rather the structural impossibility of language to fully satiate desire. It is the name for the absence of a signifier that, if present, would eradicate the difference between the subject and the other. As a messy substitute for this gap, a surplus enjoyment emerges in its place; it is this surplus enjoyment that is given the name of sex within psychoanalysis. Following this line of argumentation, it is wrong to conceive of sex as a natural force repressed by improper language. Instead, it must be understood as the very product of the subject's entrance into discourse and into contact with the other. There is no freedom from sexual repression: the fantasy that such an escape can be made from sexuality underwrites the discourse of the university. The fantasy that one can escape from repression requires the repression of the nature of sex itself. *Scientia Sexualis* cannot offer freedom from sexuality but only perpetual confession both vocal and performative. In the compulsion to repeat these practices, in the perpetual incitement to speak and act one's sexual truth, that antagonistic element of sexuality, the drive, can be perceived because no matter how precise, how honest, the subject's discourse, something more can be said and must be said.

Another dissenting voice can be found in the correspondence with the defence counsel. Psychoanalyst Charles Rycroft was asked to testify to the publication of *Lady Chatterley* benefitting the psychoanalytic profession. In his letter, he first states his reservations about his status as an expert in regard to literary merit and goes on to dismiss the defence's claim that publication of the text would allow, for the first time, a complete psychological biography of D.H. Lawrence to be completed. Rycroft then goes on to dispute the grounds upon which the defence framed the relation between subject and text:

> Clinical experience gives no grounds for supposing an individual's moral and sexual nature can be injured by the written word, while psychoanalytical research suggests that the causes of those disturbances of behaviour which the law calls corrupt and depraved lie in the history of his relationship with people, pre-eminently those who had influence on him in his childhood and adolescence. Clinical practice also suggests that descriptions of sexual matters which are explicit are erotically less stimulating than those which are elusive and suggestive.

Rycroft's analysis of the potential effects of the literary text differs massively from the argument presented in court: there is no clinical evidence as to the harmful effects of literature; instead, Rycroft emphases the subject's relation to the other as the source of any pathological behaviour in the subject, directly contradicting the defence's argument that an improper relationship towards certain signifiers of sex could cause neurosis and that an encounter with *Lady Chatterley* could affect them in a positive manner. Rycroft also undermines with the supposition that sexuality can and should be freed by the literary text and the law: if it is the case that explicit sexual descriptions are 'erotically less stimulating than those which are elusive and suggestive', then sexuality is linked to the failure of the signified, enjoyment emerges at the site of this failure. Far from wanting to be freed by honest mimesis, sexuality emerges most strongly as it encounters the undecidable.

Rycroft's analysis is unfit for the defence's narrative. Much like in the case of Eliot, this aspect of psychiatry is more harmful than beneficial to the defence's narrative, it must then be silenced in order to give the impression of a unified and stable body of knowledge to which the defence can appeal to for a claim to truth. The very precondition to a claim to truth becomes the repression of that antagonistic element within the body of knowledge being mobilized. And it is precisely that uncooperative and unassimilable part that psychoanalysis defines as the sexual: the sexual is not the guarantor of the sexual relation but evidence of its failure, and sex is the result of the sexual non-relation. But as we have seen, the sexual is being coded as something quite different in the trial, as the sexual relation's saviour.

With the defence's strategic disavowal of this antagonistic element of sexuality, it is important to compare these accounts of sexuality to the one given in court during the trial. James Hemming, a child psychologist, was the defence's choice as expert witness from the psychiatric profession. In his testimony, the power of sex is figured not as disruptive but as cure to a process of corruption active in contemporary society:

> Today young people are subjected to a constant titillation and insinuation of what I would describe as shallow and corrupting values with regard to sex and the relationships between the sexes. [...] [A young girl is told] that if she has the right proportions, wears the right clothes, uses the right

> cosmetic she will be irresistible to men, and that is the supreme achievement of a woman. [...] [S]o far as the young man is concerned [he is taught] that sex is nothing more than a physical thrill, that to have a pretty woman in one's arms is the supreme ecstasy of life and that to seduce a woman is manly. [...] As such, the content of *Lady Chatterley's Lover* is an antidote, a positive antidote to shallow, superficial values of sex which are widely current today and which are now corrupting the attitude of young people towards sex.[84]

The discourse of corruption and the figure of the child/young-person previously mobilized for the purpose of banning a book in the name of protecting the child is used here in order to figure *Lady Chatterley's Lover* as 'an antidote' to the values Hemming perceives as corrupting children. This discourse of antidotes is also distinctly pharmacological but in a way that mirrors previous trials wherein the corruptive substance that induced isolating, harmful and untrue enjoyment was the literary text: here, the text is no longer an embodiment of the death drive but an embodiment of truth that will regenerate England's youth and teach them to enjoy in the right way. But in offering the literary text as a signifier for true sex against the false sex of consumer society, the literary text no longer holds the position of *pharmakon* but instead sex itself appears as a *pharmakon*, both poison and cure. The text is the means by which the sexual relation which, like Hoggart, Hemming understands as under threat from the market can be saved. Later, he describes the text as presenting 'the true sex relationship', and in doing so, Hemming presents a choice between the true enjoyment of the sexual relation and the 'titillation' and 'insinuation' of sex as commodity and in those terms implies a lack of substance and an element of deception in that enjoyment, an absence of truth.[85]

Entirely absent from Hemming's account is the problematic relation between sex and truth present in the other psychiatric experts' correspondence: sex, the 'real' sex of *Lady Chatterley* at least, is undoubtedly true and good. The literary text gains its legitimacy and absolves itself of the accusation of obscenity by virtue of this proximity to truth. The suspicion of the literary text that has defined these trials is eradicated on the provision that it would bring the reader closer to the truth and closer to the polis as a result. These overlapping relationships between sexuality, truth and health create a form of duty in both the literary text and the medical professional. Such a relation can be seen in Hemming's proscriptive statement that:

> [f]or young people to grow up and marry with a prudish and ashamed attitude towards sex is positively harmful. *Lady Chatterley's Lover* presents sex as it should be presented, where the relationship of sex is something joyful and exuberant, tender, playful even, and certainly mutual. I think this kind of picture entirely right.[86]

Hemming here speaks from a position of absolute knowledge as to the meaning of the text, sex and the healthiest manner in which a universal subject must relate to them. It is proscriptive of both the subject and the text's duty to that truth. The text has a duty to tell the truth, which, in another sense, is a duty to repress its own sexual aspect, that is the element which refuses to do its duty towards presenting the relations between the sexes, and the act of heterosexual sex as harmonious, fulfilling and on the side of life.

Due to the similar testimonies of dozens of expert witnesses from diverse bodies of knowledge, all testifying to the healthy effect of the text upon the subject and grounding the truth of these claims upon the legitimacy of their respective bodies of knowledge, the text was cleared of obscenity on 2 November 1960. This victory was based upon proving the effect of the text, the text's essence, was knowable, clearly demonstrated and beneficial to the public. As in the *Ulysses* trial of 1933, the text's previously perceived harmful effects were transfigured into curative properties. But there, the text was represented as a truthful depiction of modernity, and this truth value constituted its literary value. In this trial, however, it is precisely the status of *Lady Chatterley's Lover* as an anachronism, a gateway to a previous age that provides its power to potentially restore the fantasy of the sexual relation that the market, the new embodiment of the death drive, comes to represent. But in order for this truth claim to be made, as with all the truth claims about the texts made from both critic and lawyer, the text has been spoken for, strategically read and carefully reconstructed in order for that truth claim to function.

Notes

1 Giorgio Agamben, *Homo Sacer: Sovereign Power and Bare Life*, trans. Daniel Heller-Roazen, (Stanford, CA: Stanford University Press, 1998), p. 1.
2 Ibid. p. 3.
3 Ibid. p. 7.
4 There are analogies here between Agamben's forms of life and Lee Edelman's distinction between heteronormative desire and queer *jouissance*. Queer *jouissance*, for Edelman, constitutes an enjoyment of the subject's singularity, the remainder that the Symbolic order cannot code. The queer is thus included in the Symbolic through a violent exclusion of those that are coded as queer. The relation of sovereign to *homo sacer* is closely paralleled with that of child and the queer in Edelman's analysis. However, the same problems emerge in Agamben analysis as I have dealt with in my previous chapter on Lawrence in regards to Edelman: the clear distinction between these forms of life becomes much more difficult to maintain with the introduction of the signifier and the unconscious. In both theories, we are still enmeshed on the male side of Lacan's graph of sexuation; caught in the closed set of limit, transgression and repetition that Freud describes in *Totem and Taboo*.
5 *Homo Sacer* is, according to Agamben, drawing upon Roman law, a person stripped of their legal rights and exiled but also at the same time forbidden from being sacrificed. In being exiled, he is cast outside the polis, reduced to bare life. But in being regarded as sacred, evidenced in the taboo against his killing, *homo sacer* maintains a link to the law: he, like the sovereign, maintains a liminal relation to the law, both inside and outside, included and excluded.

6 The five novels in question were Katherine Dyson Taylor's *Julia*, Vivian Connell's *September in Quinze*, Walter Baxter's *The Image and the Search*, Hugh McGraw's *The Man in Control* and Stanley Kaufmann's *The Philanderer.* These prosecutions followed the same structure as the ones recounted in this thesis. Three of the five authors were American, and their prosecution is linked by David Bradshaw to rising concerns of the threat of obscene American literature (David Bradshaw, 'American Beastliness', in *Prudes on the Prowl: Fiction and Obscenity in England, 1850 to the Present Day*, ed. Rachel Potter, (Cambridge: Cambridge University Press, 2013), pp. 138–159). The figure of the Young-Girl also appears in the trial of *September in Quinze*: summing up, the Recorder of London, Sir Gerald Dodson declared that literature must be suitable for 'a callow youth, or a girl just budding into womanhood' (quoted in Ibid. p. 148). He also went on to state that prosecution was necessary 'for the youth of this nation to be protected and that the fountain of our national blood should not be polluted at its source' (Ibid. p. 148). This evident investment in the young girl as the victim of a substance that's corrupting influence could destabilize the nation is remarkably similar to the discourse of the 19th-century prosecutions almost 100 years previously.

7 Quoted in Cecil H. Rolph, *The Trial of Lady Chatterley: Regina v Penguin Books Limited*, (London: Penguin, 1990), p. xvii.

8 The Obscene Publications Act 1959, S.1 SS.1, http://www.legislation.gov.uk/ukpga/Eliz2/7-8/66/section/1, (accessed 6 June 2017).

9 The Obscene Publications Act 1959, http://www.legislation.gov.uk/ukpga/Eliz2/7-8/66/section/4/enacted, (accessed 6 July 2017).

10 Comment in John Bull 1928, in *The Critical Heritage: D.H. Lawrence*, ed. Ronald P. Draper (London: Routledge, 2002), pp. 177–179, p. 177.

11 Ibid. p. 177.

12 Ibid. p. 179.

13 Ibid.

14 Sean Matthews, 'The Trial of *Lady Chatterley's Lover*: "The Most Thorough and Expensive Seminar on Lawrence's Work Ever Given"', in *New D.H. Lawrence*, ed. Howard Booth, (Manchester: Manchester University Press, 2009), pp. 169–193, p. 169.

15 Frank R. Leavis, *Revaluation: Tradition and Development in English Poetry*, (London: Ivan R. Dee, 1998).

16 Frank R. Leavis, *D.H. Lawrence: Novelist*, (London: Pelican, 1973), p. 12.

17 Frank R. Leavis, *The Common Pursuit*, (London: Faber and Faber, 2011), p. 41.

18 Leavis, *Lawrence*, p. 14.

19 Thomas S. Eliot, *After Strange Gods: A Primer on Modern Hersey*, (London: Faber and Faber, 1934), p. 18.

20 What seems to be elided by Eliot in this passage is the potential irony of Bloom's definition of nation. To define a nation as 'the same people living in the same place' is at once a statement of the final instance of the nation that declares the final instance of what is shared, the 'blood kinship' that Eliot connects it to in this passage. But the definition also potentially undoes the ties of blood kinship between subjects in that it renders arbitrary the shared fantasies of collective identity that a tradition maintains. With this in mind, it becomes more difficult to figure Joyce as the champion of the shared values of Christianity, and Eliot's dependence upon such an ambivalent definition would also seem to put in jeopardy the ontological status of the tradition he desires to protect. The knowingly performative, or perhaps, the performance of performativity, in Joyce troubles any attempt to find a truth claim upon the text.

21 Frank R. Leavis, *The Great Tradition*, (London: Chatto & Windus, 1960), pp. 8–9.

22 The choice between life and death is reminiscent of Edelman's discussion of the figure of the child in contemporary American politics. Discussing the similarities between anti-abortion and pro-choice discourses, Edelman identifies the absence of any meaningful choice, only a reframing of the discourses around the rights of the child and the definition of life:

> Who *would*, after all, come out *for* abortion or stand *against* futurity, and so against *life?* Who would destroy the child and with it the vitalizing fantasy of bridging, in time, the gap of signification (a fantasy that distracts us from the violence of the drives while permitting us to enact them)?
>
> (Edelman, *No Future*, p. 16)

An implicit false choice is similarly enunciated in Leavis. Who would choose the literature of death over the literature of life? In Leavis, there is not so much a renunciation of obscenity, a Leavisite obscenity would be precisely this deathly allegiance to the signifier, but rather, a reframing of the canon, reallocating obscene jouissance in other texts. It is the same underlying framework as the arguments of the Society of Authors wherein it is not that obscene doesn't exist, but it's just that Lawrence's are wrongly accused. Lawrence is on the side of *bios*, it is those overly stylized writers like Flaubert and Joyce, those on the side of the signifier, on the side of the drives, that threaten life.

23 Leavis also maintained a similarly hostile relation to Joyce throughout his writing, attributing the same life-denying sentiment to his writing. In *The Great Tradition*, *Ulysses* is 'a dead end, or at least a pointer to disintegration' (Ibid. p. 26). The same accusation is levelled at the work of Henry Miller and Djuna Barnes. These authors, under the influence of Joyce and championed by Eliot, are representative of 'a desire, in a Lawrentian phrase, to "do dirt" on life' (Ibid. p. 26). Much like Eliot's description of tradition was dependent upon a citation from Joyce, here, Leavis appropriates Lawrence's discourse to distinguish between those texts on the side of life and those against it. This dependency of the critic upon their object of study to justify their own position betrays a fundamental tautological instability in their claim to objectivity.

Although there is no stated desire to ban these authors, it is telling that, in the cases of Flaubert, Joyce and Miller, these texts were tried for obscenity on the grounds of their immorality. The moral categories of Leavisite discourse repeat the preceding discourse's tendency to delegate opposing forms of enjoyment: in Leavis, they are the enjoyment of life and the enjoyment of death. The texts that are representative of the tradition change in Leavis, but the structure of the discourse centred on an empty signifier remains. We are not then dealing with the introduction of a new emancipatory mode of reading, but rather, a refiguring of power relations that allow for the introduction of Lawrence, and by extension working-class culture, into a discourse that had previously excluded them.

24 Quoted in Leavis, *Tradition*, p. 8.

25 Leavis, *Lawrence*, p. 72.

26 Ibid. p. 129.

27 Ibid. p. 42.

28 Jacques Derrida, 'Signature, Event, Context', in *Limited Inc.*, (Evanston, IL: Northwestern University Press, 1988), pp. 1–25, p. 12.

29 My own citation of Derrida is implicated in this double play of citation. The context of Derrida's words in his essay is lost, and those words find a new context in my own argument towards my own truth claims. Citation is, as Derrida and Lacan attest to in their own registers, the condition of signification itself, and even in a critique of mastery, a certain control and violence must be performed. Where my discourse differs from that of the master, I hope, is the absence of a claim to a truth that is self-evident.

30 Geoff Bucher, 'Bureaucratic Speech Acts and the University Discourse: Lacan's Theory of Modernity', in *Jacques Lacan and the Other Side of Psychoanalysis: Reflections on Seminar XVII*, ed. Justin Clemens and Russell Grigg, (London: Duke University Press, 2006), pp. 274–292, p. 279.

31 Shoshana Felman and Dori Laub, *Testimony: Crises of Witnessing in Literature, Psychoanalysis, and History*, (London: Routledge, 1992), p. 3.

32 The same dynamic can be seen in the Leavisite demand that literature bear witness to life: as that outside the signifier, the stuff that the signifier tries to attach itself to and

colonize. Life resists its own telling and in performing such resistance attains its value. Eliot, in a reading, I will return to later, in this chapter, focuses on life's recalcitrance to the signifier by noting that Lawrence's obsession with Life was bound to transform into an obsession with death. To subject life to the signifier is to negate what makes it valuable in the first place: in this failure, however, the fantasy object of life increases in desirability. Very quickly, *bios* can turn to *zoe*, purity into obscenity.

33 Ibid. p. 3.
34 Richard Hoggart, *The Uses of Literature: Aspects of Working Class Life*, (London: Penguin, 2009), p. 30.
35 Ibid. p. 32.
36 Ibid. p. 31.
37 Ibid. p. 202.
38 Ibid. p. 37.
39 A tension emerges here that is not quite worked out during the trial: the literary text is figured as a form of resistance to the forces of the market that seek to commodify all aspects of modern life. However, the means by which this resistance can take place is a legal battle for the right to publish and sell the text which will in turn, according to this argument, resist its own commodification. The temptation here is to accuse these authors and critics of hypocrisy or bad faith in their arguments. But rather, I wish to argue that it is fantasy that is operative here, a fantasy of a return to a prelapsarian state of authentic and whole enjoyment. The market is thus the agent of the split between the true work of art and its simulacrum, the 'confetti literature' that Hoggart disparages. But this fantasy functions as a screen for a much more disturbing truth: the split cannot be located in a certain time or attributed to any agent; it is constitutive of language itself. In this way, the arguments of Hoggart and Leavis against consumer capitalism help to encourage the ever widening commodification of the literary and the sexual whilst purporting to resist it.

   It is a displacement of the initial accusation towards literature. It was before the literary text that was the bearer of non-being and destructive jouissance. Leavis and Hoggart assert that it is the market that is the agent of this destructive force. Both forms presuppose a unitary, good and healthy society at risk from various embodiments of the death drive. This movement represents a reversal of the moral categories but not a radical break.
40 Ibid. p. 133.
41 David H. Lawrence, *A Propos of Lady Chatterley's Lover*, in *Lady Chatterley's Lover*, (London: Penguin, 2001), p. 307.
42 Rolph, *The Trial of Lady Chatterley*, p. 11.
43 Ibid. p. 35.
44 Rachel Bowlby, *Shopping with Freud*, (London: Routledge, 1993), p. 25.
45 Gérard Wajcman, *The Hysteric's Discourse*, http://www.lacan.com/hystericdiscf.htm, (accessed 20 June 2017).
46 Ibid.
47 Lacan, *Seminar XVII*, (London: Norton, 2008), p. 183.
48 Ibid. p. 185.
49 Ibid. p. 189.
50 Ibid. p. 15.
51 Ibid. p. 77.
52 Ibid. p. 188.
53 Ibid. pp. 104–105.
54 Ibid. p. 148.
55 In *Society Must Be Defended*, Foucault makes a similar point when he describes the discourse of history as 'the uninterrupted ode in which power perpetuate[s] itself' (Foucault, *Society*, p. 70). The knowledge of the past that is produced in history conforms to, confirms and celebrates as a moral good, the contemporary master signifier

from which it comes. In this way, any given discourse of truth can become 'an operator of power, an intensifier of power' (Ibid. p. 68). The same function I wish to ascribe to the discourse of literary criticism during this trial. The defence of *Lady Chatterley's Lover* constitutes an ode to life and, as such, a valorization of biopolitical domination.

56 Bruce Fink, *The Lacanian Subject: Between Language and Jouissance*, (Princeton, NJ: Princeton University Press, 1995), pp. 132–133.

57 There is a link here to *Totem and Taboo* once again. The civilization set up by the sons of the primal father is founded only after the father's murder, the failure of the master. It is on the condition of his failure that the sons come to identify with the father to see in him their truth. In his failure, the father is reinstated to the level of master, and it is in his name that the laws of the culture are based. Freud's myth, then, performs the same transition from master to university that is apparent in the *Lady Chatterley* trial.

58 Frank R. Leavis, *The Spectator*, 17 February 1961, p. 13.

59 Passages from *D.H. Lawrence: Novelist* are to be found in the defence's briefing notes in the Penguin Archives at Bristol.

60 Thomas S. Eliot, *The Letters of T. S. Eliot Volume 6: 1932–1933*, (London: Faber and Faber, 2016), p. 584. In the same letter, Eliot explains his aversion to *Lolita*:

> it seemed to me a book which would make anyone in which such a perverse tendency was latent more conscious of his craving. And it seems to me a peculiarly undesirable book at a time when so many little girls have been abducted and strangled. [...] I only read *Lolita* because I had read about it and wanted to see how it compared to my mind with *Lady Chatterley's Lover*. And it did seem to me that the latter book came out as something very much more decent.
>
> (Ibid. p. 584)

The haphazard dissemination of the signifier and its corrupting effects on the potential reader that characterized the previous prosecution of texts for obscenity are prevalent in Eliot's analysis of *Lolita*, even in the sense that his concern is for the protection of the Young-Girl: but whereas others had worried about the potentially damaging effects of the signifier in corrupting the Young-Girl directly, here it is a corruption done by proxy, by those already corrupted and helped into knowledge of their own evil through the text. It is also worth noting that the virtue of Lawrence's text, its value as literature, is only revealed when placed into contrast with Nabokov's. Much like Eliot's description of tradition in *Tradition and the Individual Talent*, the emergence of a new text changes the appreciation of the texts that come before, even if that text is subsequently abjected.

61 Sabine Spielrein, 'Destruction as The Cause of Coming into Being', in *Journal of Analytical Psychology*, Vol. 39, 1994, pp. 155–186, p. 157.

62 Eliot, *After Strange Gods*, p. 61.

63 Ibid.

64 Ibid.

65 Roberto Esposito, *Bios: Biopolitics and Philosophy*, trans Timothy Campbell, (London: University of Minnesota Press, 2008), p. 47.

66 Ibid. pp. 44–45.

67 Ibid. p. 45.

68 Eric Santner, *The Royal Remains: The People's Two Bodies and the Endgames of Sovereignty*, (London: University of Chicago Press, 2011), p. 21.

69 Foucault, *The History of Sexuality Vol I*, p. 112.

70 Ibid. p. 25.

71 Michel Foucault, 'Preface to Transgression', in *Language, Counter-Memory, Practice: Selected Interviews*, ed. and trans. Donald F. Bouchard, (Ithaca, NY: Cornell University Press, 1977), pp. 29–52, pp. 29–30.

72 Zupančič, *Sex?*, p. 3.

73 Copjec, *Desire*, p. 209.

74 Zupančič, *Sex?*, p. 39.
75 Foucault flirts with this interpretation of psychoanalysis in both *The History of Madness* and *The History of Sexuality*. He remains ambivalent, however, as can be seen in his discussion of psychoanalysis in *The Order of Things*.
76 Lacan, quoted in Zupancic, *Sex?*, p. 41.
77 Zupančič, *Sex?*, p. 43.
78 Ibid.
79 Ibid. p. 35.
80 Matthews, *Lady Chatterley's Lover*, p. 171.
81 David H. Lawrence, *Lady Chatterley's Lover*, (London: Penguin, 2011), p. 103.
82 Ibid.
83 Sigmund Freud, 'Repression', in *The Standard Edition of The Complete Works of Sigmund Freud Volume XIV, (1914–1916)*, trans. James Strachey, (London: Hogarth, 1957), pp. 141–158.
84 Rolph, *The Trial of Lady Chatterley*, p. 118.
85 Ibid.
86 Ibid. p. 119.

Bibliography

Agamben, Giorgio, *Homo Sacer: Sovereign Power and Bare Life*, trans. Daniel Heller-Roazen, (Stanford, CA: Stanford University Press, 1998).

Bowlby, Rachel, *Shopping with Freud*, (London: Routledge, 1993).

Bradshaw, David, 'American Beastliness', in *Prudes on the Prowl: Fiction and Obscenity in England, 1850 to the Present Day*, ed. Rachel Potter, (Cambridge: Cambridge University Press, 2013), pp. 138–159.

Bucher, Geoff, 'Bureaucratic Speech Acts and the University Discourse: Lacan's Theory of Modernity', in *Jacques Lacan and the Other Side of Psychoanalysis: Reflections on Seminar XVII*, ed. Justin Clemens and Russell Grigg, (London: Duke University Press, 2006), pp. 274–291.

Copjec, Joan, *Read My Desire*, (London: MIT Press, 1994).

Derrida, Jacques, 'Signature, Event, Context', in *Limited Inc.*, (Evanston, IL: Northwestern University Press, 1988), pp. 1–25.

Draper, Ronald P. (ed.), *The Critical Heritage: D.H. Lawrence*, (London: Routledge, 2002).

Eliot, Thomas S., *After Strange Gods: A Primer on Modern Hersey*, (London: Faber and Faber, 1934).

———, *The Letters of T. S. Eliot Volume 6: 1932–1933*, (London: Faber and Faber, 2016).

Esposito, Roberto, *Bios: Biopolitics and Philosophy*, trans. Timothy Campbell, (London: University of Minnesota Press, 2008).

Felman, Shoshana, *Testimony: Crises of Witnessing in Literature, Psychoanalysis, and History*, (London: Routledge, 1992).

Fink, Bruce, *The Lacanian Subject: Between Language and Jouissance*, (Princeton, NJ: Princeton University Press, 1995).

Foucault, Michel, *The History of Sexuality Volume I: The Will to Knowledge*, trans. Robert Hurley, (London: Random House, 1988).

———, 'Preface to Transgression', in *Language, Counter-Memory, Practice: Selected Interviews*, ed. and trans. Donald F. Bouchard, (Ithaca, NY: Cornell University Press, 1977), pp. 52–59.

Hoggart, Richard, *The Uses of Literature: Aspects of Working Class Life*, (London: Penguin, 2009).

Lacan, Jacques, *Seminar XVII*, (London: Norton, 2008).
Lawrence, David H., *Lady Chatterley's Lover*, (London: Penguin, 2011).
———, *A Propos of Lady Chatterley's Lover*, in *Lady Chatterley's Lover*, (London: Penguin, 2001), pp. 289–322.
Leavis, Frank R., *The Common Pursuit*, (London: Faber and Faber, 2011), p. 41.
———, *D.H. Lawrence: Novelist*, (London: Pelican, 1973).
———, *The Great Tradition*, (London: Chatto & Windus, 1960).
———, Letter in *The Spectator*, 17 February 1961.
———, *Revaluation: Tradition and Development in English Poetry*, (London: Ivan R. Dee, 1998).
Matthews, Sean, 'The Trial of *Lady Chatterley's Lover*: "The Most through and Expensive Seminar on Lawrence's Work Ever Given"', in *New D.H Lawrence*, ed. Howard Booth, (Manchester: Manchester University Press, 2009), pp. 169–193.
Rolph, Cecil H., *The Trial of Lady Chatterley: Regina v. Penguin Books Limited*, (London: Penguin, 1990).
Santner, Eric, *The Royal Remains: The People's Two Bodies and the Endgames of Sovereignty*, (London: University of Chicago Press, 2011).
Wajcman, Gérard, *The Hysteric's Discourse*, http://www.lacan.com/hystericdiscf.htm.
Zupančič, Alenka, *What Is Sex?* (London: MIT Press, 2017).

CONCLUSION

All of the trials I have discussed in this book present themselves as a choice between two forms of fantasy, one is the form of fantasy that is coded as isolating the subject from the truth, the fantasy that intoxicates the subject with the enjoyment of untruth and death; the other form of fantasy is the shared fantasy of truth that facilitates the beginning and maintenance of a shared identity between subjects. One name for the shared fantasy towards which the law works is the sexual relation, and, tellingly, it is to sex that these trials constantly return, with the law seeking to define its meaning, its proper uses and presentation. All of this work is done in the name of the sexual relation and against those other fantasies that challenge and threaten its consistency.

These competing forms of fantasy are not self-forming and self-preserving. As I have worked to show, the maintenance of collective fantasies of truth requires considerable labour on the part of both subjects and social institutions such as the law and the university. Neither is the meaning of the objects that are invested with fantasmatic content also stable, they too can change according to the necessary demands of the maintenance of the fantasy. The literary text, and by extension the names of Joyce and Lawrence, are themselves an example of these shifting investments, at one time figured as a threat to the fantasy of the sexual relation, and ultimately co-opted as its saviour. In each of these interpretations of the object, a part of the object's being is necessarily repressed in the name of the sexual relation. Each trial in this book can thus be understood as a crisis in this fantasy, a queering of the master signifiers upon which the sexual relation is maintained: the name, the Young-Girl, medicine and sex. In each trial, the investments in these signifiers came under scrutiny and though the legal decision ended this crisis by declaring the truth of the text, the work required to

DOI: 10.4324/9781003202509

legitimate that decision stands as its own form of testimony to the fantasmatic investments operative within the law and the culture in which those laws govern.

But like the critics and lawyers who must necessarily repress certain aspects of the text in order to produce its truth, this text, too, is implicated in that procedure. By choosing only the trials of Joyce and Lawrence, I have omitted a vast number of other texts, both canonical and marginal, that were tried for obscenity after both the 1933 and 1960 trials which were coded as embodiments of the death drive just as the previous trials of *Ulysses* and *The Rainbow* had done. But the choice of trials and omission of others is instructive if not comprehensive. The narrative presented in this book, from literature as embodiment of the death drive towards literature as a catalyst for cultural regeneration, serves as a means to interrogate the manner in which legal and academic institutions interpret and claim the truth of the literary text, and how these truth claims reproduce and maintain wider cultural investments and power structures.

To continue past 1960 and the manner in which the embodiments of obscenity shift from the literary text onto other mediums and technologies, from video to the internet, would also further complicate the underlying thesis of this text. This historical moment also witnesses the beginning of a shift in power formations; Liberalism is beginning to give way to neoliberalism, anxiety about market forces allowing unfettered access to the dangerous *jouissance* of the drive increases amongst left leaning literary critics and decrease within culture at large. An analysis of obscenity in the late 20th century would need to be more attuned to the market as *pharmakon*, a status only briefly broached in the final chapter of this work. The combination of a transition between power structures and increasing technological production creates a new regime of truth, a regime whose parameters are far more difficult to discern than the regime analysed throughout this book. Buse succinctly details this shift when he notes that the digital regime of truth, our contemporary episteme, is an era in which 'both the Master's and the University discourse have suffered serial erosions, with mastery and knowledge de-supposed by information and electronic storage'.[1] Another history of obscenity more attuned to the development and problematics of *techne* could be written that would be able to trace the drift of *jouissance* over media throughout this period and beyond. Again, this book has acknowledged and skirted around this alternative approach but has not explored it in the detail it deserves.

Instead, this book has chosen the literary text as the basis for its analysis, partly because of the sustained surveillance it was subject to over the years detailed in these chapters, but, also, because of the cultural and personal investments that the literary text represents. The literary text both refuses to accede to the law's demands for truth but also, through this silence, is spoken for and made to work in the name of multiple different forms of power. A close reading of the trials, as I hope to have demonstrated, manifests the degree to which these appropriations of the text, the fixing of its truth, require a large amount of labour on the part of the law and critics. The trials themselves give witness to the process by which the text's truth is constructed whilst also leaving an excess, traces of those parts of the text left behind. In another sense, these trials, read in conjunction with one another, are also testimony to the power of the text's silence, a silence that refuses to comply with the law's demands and signifies the fundamental resistance of the literary text to both the law and literary criticism's desire.

Note

1 Peter Buse, 'On the Diagonal: Jacques Lacan's Reading Lists', in *Parallax*, Vol. 22, No. 4, p. 483.

INDEX